CARE AT HOME FOR PEOPLE LIVING WITH DEMENTIA

Delaying Institutionalization, Sustaining Families

Christine Ceci and Mary Ellen Purkis

With a foreword by
Jeannette Pols

First published in Great Britain in 2023 by

Policy Press, an imprint of
Bristol University Press
University of Bristol
1-9 Old Park Hill
Bristol
BS2 8BB
UK
t: +44 (0)117 374 6645
e: bup-info@bristol.ac.uk

Details of international sales and distribution partners are available at
policy.bristoluniversitypress.co.uk

British Library Cataloguing in Publication Data
A catalogue record for this book is available from the British Library

ISBN 978-1-4473-5928-9 hardcover
ISBN 978-1-4473-5929-6 paperback
ISBN 978-1-4473-5930-2 ePub
ISBN 978-1-4473-5931-9 ePdf

Cover design: Andrew Corbett
Front cover image: Rita Sirignano

Bristol University Press and Policy Press use environmentally responsible
print partners.

Printed in Great Britain by CPI Group (UK) Ltd, Croydon, CR0 4YY

FSC
www.fsc.org
MIX
Paper | Supporting
responsible forestry
FSC® C013604

Contents

About the authors

Christine Ceci, PhD, RN, is Associate Professor in the Faculty of Nursing at the University of Alberta, Canada. Her programme of research includes empirical and theoretical work concerned with the organization of care practices for frail older people, currently focused on the situations of families in which one member has a diagnosis of dementia. She co-edited, with Mary Ellen Purkis and Kristin Björnsdóttir, *Perspectives on Care at Home for Older People* (Routledge, 2011) and *Philosophy of Nursing: 5 Questions* with Anette Forss and John Drummond (Automatic Press, 2013). She is a collaborator in the Care Practices Research Network (www.ualberta.ca/nursing/research/research-units/care-practice-research-network).

Mary Ellen Purkis, PhD, is Professor Emerita in the School of Nursing at the University of Victoria, Canada. For nearly 30 years Mary Ellen has conducted ethnographic fieldwork in the area of home-based care. Increasingly, such care focuses on the health and social concerns of older adults. Her research interests have focused primarily on care at home as this intersects with professional practices of organizing.

Acknowledgements

Our pathway towards writing this book has been supported by many good colleagues who have engaged in these questions about care and practices over many decades. This particular project began in 2014, and here we acknowledge the funding of our work by the Canadian Institute of Health Research (CIHR, MOP 133462) whose support made all the ensuing activities possible. Central to this work, we share our deep gratitude to the four families who opened their homes and experiences to us, generously giving of their time and stories. We also acknowledge the contributions of the many other participants in this research. These were our 'key informants' – health service managers, programme coordinators, frontline workers – committed and deeply concerned individuals serving within the governmental, non-governmental and voluntary care sectors. We also thank all those who participated in our film discussion groups, broadening and deepening our understanding of the questions that shaped our research.

Although we have together been exploring practices organizing home care in Western Canada for many years, this work has been vastly enhanced through collaboration with talented colleagues from many locations – both fellow academics and students. Heather Stanley, a postdoctoral fellow, joined the project in the early days, working to elaborate the historical and current context of the work. Holly Symonds-Brown joined as a new doctoral student, bringing significant and singular insight to our understanding of the problems facing families. Harkeert Judge, also a doctoral student, brought her curiosity and enthusiasm for learning to all our discussions. Both contributed significantly to the development of our film, developing scenes and dialogue, managing people and locations, as well as taking on acting roles (!) – this part of the project could definitely not have been accomplished without them.

Academic colleagues have also been vital. Kristin Björnsdóttir has long been a strong collaborator on our path of learning about home care practices. Jeannette Pols and Ingunn Moser deepened our appreciation for care practices, how to study them, how to write about them, how they interact and grow and sometimes, just as suddenly, stop – and why starting and stopping and everything in between is so important to follow. In 2016, this group of scholars, their students and colleagues, gathered in Reykjavík to take some time out of everyday academic life to think in depth about care practices. Our colleagues

v

Isabela Cancio Velloso and Meiriele Tavares Araujo joined us from Brazil and shared the work they were doing there examining good home care practices. Bernike Pasveer joined us from the Netherlands and asked us questions that made us think more about technologies, caring and ageing. A year later, many of this group met again in Vallendar, Germany, this time invited by Helen Kohlen and there, our Care Practices Research Network took on a more formal character. With thanks to our younger colleagues – in particular, Holly Symonds-Brown and Harkeert Judge – who know how to practise in the space of social media, we created a presence on Twitter (@CarePractices), and our network continues to grow as a result!

This is a story of networks that grow outwards, finding people who ask interesting questions about care and practicing that we have gained so much from over our years of colleagueship mixed so happily with friendship. But networks closer to home also engaged in sustaining practices that contributed to this book. Here, we thank our families for surrounding us with practices of care that freed us to think, talk and write together. For Mary Ellen, there is her sister Karen – chef extraordinaire – and her father Jack – ever-reliable pet sitter. For Christine there is, as always, Joe – patient, kind and always willing to be 'first listener' of sometimes bumpy drafts.

All of these actors (and more) are inextricably part of the stories we share here. We thank them all – for their support during this long period when we were utterly distracted by this task at hand.

Foreword

Jeannette Pols

What is the problem with dementia? We have heard many messages that there *is* an urgent problem with dementia. There are metaphors of tsunamis of ageing people developing forgetfulness, and statistics predicting the size of this tsunami. Strategies are developed to promote 'ageing in place', that is, to care for people at home, so as not to flood institutions and make healthcare costs explode. Millions of dollars, euros and yens are spent on research to find the cure for Alzheimer's disease, as well as to develop the technologies that will accommodate the care for the increasing amount of people already suffering from it. And there are ink-black stories about the great fear for Alzheimer's disease as the exemplification of losing one's humanity: a loss of cognition, autonomy and control over one's bowels and bladder. This 'fourth age imaginary' predicts a 'sailing into darkness' of what was once a human subject (Driessen, 2019).

These are 'loud' stories, the authors of this book claim. They scream alarm and collapse, but their understanding of 'the problem of dementia' is at the same time very diverse. The problem of dementia, this book argues, is, paradoxically, both overdetermined and underdefined. Christine Ceci and Mary Ellen Purkis add a quieter story, one that may take some more concentrated listening, but that digs deeper when one wants to get a grip on what the problem with dementia might be and what kind of help might relieve it. The book focuses on the problem of sustaining families at home, in order to delay institutionalization. It does so with another paradox: these are common problems, but they are not the same problems for everyone. Ceci and Purkis want to know what the 'problems of dementia', plural, become, when regarding them from amidst the very different practices through which they are addressed and lived. They side with four families living at home, and accompany them on their visits to formal caregivers. By sharing their lives, they get the 'inside view' of what it means to live with dementia at home, how the problems shift and are handled, and how formal care organizations try to help.

The focus on everyday practices does not necessarily make things easier. What becomes clear is that families seek to find help that fits their specific situation and the specific problems they are facing at a certain point in time. This can be about 'respite care' to have a break for the caring spouse from being on the alert 24/7. But it is also a life full of insolvable comparisons of possibilities and impossibilities, hopes and wishes that cannot be smoothly aligned. For instance, the book describes the case of a man who is prone to accidents of falling. The formal care system tells the family they have to prevent this at all costs. But they live in a house with many small stairs that do not accommodate a walking frame or a wheelchair. If the couple moved to a walker-friendly house, their two sons could not live with them anymore – and they are providing a large part of the care and supervision. This allows the partner to keep her outside activities. In another case, the day programme for the husband stops from day one to the next, without any suggestion for an alternative, leaving the wife in despair, calling in vain to other formal care providers who just did not happen to be there at the time she needed them. One husband works so hard to keep his wife in shape that he is nearing exhaustion, and his long letters to his doctor are an increasingly desperate call for help that does not come.

But the book does not stop with listing the specificities of familial miseries. It meticulously theorizes how we might think about these complexities, and how they may be relieved. Ceci and Purkis conceptualize the relationships between family life and formal care as 'practices *among* practices'. Relating formal care to informal care at home, they argue, too often implies overlaying the general frameworks and coherences that institutions use onto the shifting and unpredictable relations of a family at home. Formal caregivers use general concepts such as 'trajectories', biomedical understandings of dementia, and stages of dementia, but these concepts do not seamlessly fit the problems the families see for themselves. These categories provide possibilities for making cases and coherences that allow for acting. But these interventions are also standardized, by focusing their activities on what they had defined in advance to be 'the problem', and hence what help would be appropriate. This may relate for better or for worse to the particular mess of everyday life the families find themselves confronted with.

The message of the book on 'What to do?' is an important and urgent one. The authors make a plea for formal caregivers to engage in border work, work that understands that there are differences in logics and problem definitions between formal and informal care, between *this* situation at home, and the problems for which *they* have help on offer. It demands a care policy that accommodates care for *specificities*, which seems all the more urgent for care that concerns everyday life, with problems that shift and do not go away, but are likely to deteriorate.

This is very different from, say, the treatment of a broken bone, where the problem can be narrowly defined and adequate help can be clearly designed. Hence, professionals caring for lives with dementia need to be provided space to think about how to collaborate with situations that are different, specific, and most probably divergent from what they formally have on offer. Rather than a coordination of fixed services, the authors suggest thinking about care for dementia within a *patchwork* of care provisions, where different fabrics of problems, needs and arrangements are linked together by using different kinds of stitches. This invites formal care providers to become masters at improvising and finding ways to get to the patches the families need. This can support the improvisations that families already try to make, carving out new and custom-size pathways rather than merely imposing pre-given trajectories. This demands an open mind for understanding what actually *is* the problem, and to think of a variety of possible solutions as to what might be done about it.

In a wider perspective the book poses the question of what kind of dementia we actually want to live with, and how we may do that well. This is a most urgent question that the Western world has been shying away from for too long, hiding behind the promises and financing of anti-Alzheimer drugs (with the dream of preventing it) and of new technologies to manage the grey tsunamis. The book shows that single-definition problems are doomed to fail in relation to problems that know so many specificities. It demands more rather than fewer arrangements of people, things and institutions, as elaborations of the patchwork available to people to find their pathways. It demands variety and imagination on how to make a life with dementia at home as good as possible.

Preface

This is a book about care practices that become part of people's homes when at least one person living there begins to experience cognitive decline. The book pays close attention to these practices and describes them in detail – in part to find and consider reasons why patterns among those practices may be enacted in quite different kinds of homes and at different times, as well as to be provoked by those practices that are entirely unique. Our interests in care practices leads us to try to show how they work to help people living with dementia stay at home, for a time at least.

A book that focuses on care practices is also a book that relies on the stories that people tell about their lives. When a family member lives with a diagnosis of dementia, care must be ready at all times of the day and the night to support that person in living at home. Sometimes care practices are readied ahead of time, guiding the person living with dementia, limiting the full range of options to just a few that can be managed by family members. At other times, care practices must be improvised in the moment as new possibilities arise in the midst of other life events. We could not have written about the 'thickness' (Savransky, 2018, p 217) of these problems of living at home without the generous participation of the four families whose stories were shared with us and that we describe in some detail in the chapters of this book. We thank them for their generosity and for their caring.

Living with dementia, caring for a family member who has been assigned this diagnosis, involves mutual effort sustained over a long time. We knew of other books that had been written about this life that families lead when they are caring for someone diagnosed with dementia and how many of them, focusing without necessarily foregrounding this issue of sustaining, describe this life in order to advise readers how to live well while doing this work – how to sustain themselves as caregivers. Often those instructions on how to sustain the work of caregiving come in the form of finding ways of taking time away from the work. But this is to effect a separation in caring practices that, in our book, we work to approximate in partial connection. We interrogate those connections in an attempt at provoking thinking about just what might be involved in sustaining families at home who care for a family member diagnosed with dementia.

Our interests in the field of care practices and particularly as those take shape in the context of caring for people diagnosed with dementia at home are shaped by a longer-term research focus on the work of nurses and others who practise in the community and who, historically, have brought healthcare to people living at home with chronic illnesses. The work of these nurses is often overlooked. When compared with the work of healthcare conducted in hospitals, home care nursing may appear quite mundane. And yet, the efforts of these nurses to sustain a healthcare system mostly thought of as being located in large, expensive institutions, seemed to us worthy of greater attention.

Beginning our ethnographic work of exploring the practices of home care nurses in the early 1990s meant that we have been able to trace the evolution of those caring practices from what was a practice that followed (mostly) older adults living with chronic illnesses for years, assisting those older people along the way with changes in medication, treatments and devices that might make everyday life a little easier – to practices that now are, for nurses at least, much more administrative and managerially oriented and often enacted with individuals over a much shorter period of time. When we first started following home care nurses in the early 1990s, they were being directed by their managers to find ways to get people they had been working with for many years 'off service'. Their practice now was to be much more targeted, all the easier to measure and monitor by managers working at a distance. Now, 30 years later, those nurses have, in many cases, become the managers themselves. As case managers they oversee the care trajectory of sometimes hundreds of people, some of whom are checked on once a year to assess changes in ability to live 'safely' at home. Others are monitored more frequently, mediated through the work of care aides, home support workers and others who visit people at home in carefully measured time allocations to undertake very specific tasks such as helping someone take a shower, get dressed or undressed, or take their medication.

These changes in the way healthcare in the home plays out has meant that family members have been drawn into the everyday care of their family members in ways that were not as evident 30 years ago – although, of course, families have always been engaged in caring for one another. But now that care has become something of an organizational imperative for healthcare systems. Families are seen as critical 'team members' even if the respect and regard for their contributions is not always fully appreciated. What has been recognized by senior healthcare managers, policy-makers and politicians is that *sustaining* those families so that they continue to carry a significant portion of the care required by older adults as they 'age in place' has become a policy priority.

Without adequate interrogation and an interest in examining the 'history of the present' of dementia care at home, this effort to sustain families to undertake a significant amount of unpaid work might be understood as something achieved largely by senior healthcare managers through the development and implementation of policies designed to offer targeted supports to families – particularly in the face of newer challenges associated with what is called the 'global epidemic' of dementia. As such, the everyday work of families would continue to be disregarded, and the practices they learn, developed to suit their circumstances and then improvised upon day in and day out as they conduct everyday life when someone in the family has a diagnosis of dementia, would remain invisible behind the doors and windows of those homes. In this book, and with the intellectual support of a broad network of colleagues, we set out to describe, in order to better understand (Latour, 1990), the practices involved in sustaining families engaged in caring for a family member at home who has been diagnosed with dementia.

Christine Ceci, Calgary, AB
Mary Ellen Purkis, Victoria, BC
12 February 2021

1

Studying family care practices

> Making a situation, past or present, be of importance, means
> intensifying the sense of possibles it harbours, as expressed
> by the struggles and claims to another way of making it exist.
>
> Stengers, 2017

We start this book in a 'traditional' way, outlining the 'problem of
dementia' as it is commonly thought to exist, and as it frequently
appears in policy documents – a strategy that provided a convincing
and familiar rationale for our study. What follows here constitutes, in
some sense, the 'facts' of the matter, defining a context that works to
make dementia, in its many manifestations, a matter of strategic concern
for health service planners and policy-makers. So to begin somewhat
starkly, a familiar argument goes like this.

In Canada, as in many nations, population ageing is accelerating,
and with this trend there is an increased prevalence of chronic diseases
such as dementia. The need to provide responsive care services for
older Canadians, particularly those living with Alzheimer's disease and
other dementias, is arguably the biggest challenge in healthcare policy
and practice today. Alzheimer's disease and other dementias are among
the most feared problems of ageing (CIHR, 2013, 2017; Lock, 2013;
Latimer, 2018), as well as being the most significant cause of disability
in those over the age of 65, placing a 'long-term progressive burden'
on those who care for them (Dudgeon, 2010, p 3). It is estimated
that 500,000 Canadians are living with dementia, a number that is
anticipated to increase to over one million as the population ages over
the next 25 years.

Currently, more than half of those diagnosed with a dementia are living
at home with family and community support. By 2038, this proportion
will increase to 62 per cent, or approximately 510,000 Canadians living
at home with moderate to severe cognitive impairments (Dudgeon,
2010). With more people living at home, the need for home-based
care will increase, and it is primarily family carers who will provide
this critical care to family members. It is clear, then, that family carers

make, and will continue to make, through their practices of supporting daily life with dementia, a substantial contribution to the overall sustainability of health and social care systems. Adequate support for family carers is thus considered essential to minimize risks to their health, to prevent premature institutionalization or poor care for those living with dementia, as well as to sustain the effective functioning of health and social care systems (CIHI, 2010).

This is one story, and it is a powerful one that demands attention as well as action. Demographic and epidemiological changes have led to what is often described as a crisis: burgeoning care needs, constrained public resources and insufficient support for families collide as frail older people come to be seen as an expensive problem for health and social care systems, a situation even more pronounced in the case of those living with dementia. In a worldwide response, organizations such as the World Health Organization (WHO) and the Organisation for Economic Co-operation and Development (OECD), as well as governments of individual nations and the advocacy and professional associations located therein, have argued that the sustainability of systems requires shifting care to home settings as a linchpin of health and social care policy (see, for example, Dudgeon, 2010; CIHI, 2011; WHO, 2012, 2018; CIHR, 2013, 2017; OECD, 2015, 2018; Alzheimer Society of Canada, 2016; Samus et al, 2018; NIA, 2019). Indeed, it has become a near universal policy priority that care for people living with dementia be provided in home settings for as long as possible, with this work of delaying institutionalization to be largely delegated to families (Moise et al, 2004; DH, 2009; Keefe, 2011; WHO, 2012; Walsh et al, 2020). And as Walsh and her colleagues observe (2020), this policy aim dominates in almost all nations despite a wide variance across countries in the formal services available to support people living with dementia and their families.

We note that in this story, wherein dementia figures as a crisis of epidemic proportions, 'care' features primarily in terms of its economic implications (Latimer, 2018), and the necessity of shifting care to home settings is mostly taken for granted, a kind of 'natural' solution to a problem thus posed, although the anticipated care 'burden' represented by people living with dementia for families is also of concern. In the absence of a cure, a key system response will be to manage costs by keeping people at home for as long as possible, and central to this, to keep family carers going. But in this story it is worries about the projected costs of care that seem to make dementia a pressing policy issue as if, as Latimer (2018, p 840) points out, the 'crisis' we are being asked to face is that 'we cannot afford dementia'.

It is important to observe here that our present policy conundrum, and its framing, is in no way new. Since the last part of the 20th century the attention of health policy-makers globally has increasingly been centred on the 'financial burden' of providing health and welfare services, in particular for older people, and the 'economic problem' thus represented by changing demographics (Ceci et al, 2012; Lloyd, 2012; Dalmer, 2019). And while home has always been an important site of care for sick or frail family members, since the 1990s two features of the Canadian context emerged to redefine the positioning of care at home in the 'continuum of care' as well as establishing how this issue would be addressed in policy.

First is what was repeatedly described as the 'enormous challenge' posed by the growing number of older people to the sustainability of both long-term residential care and acute care health systems (Federal/Provincial/Territorial Working Group on Home Care, 1990). Second is the fervent preoccupation with fiscal imperatives and what are often described as escalating costs in the provision of health services generally. Together these determined a key policy strategy of deinstitutionalization with a devolution of care and responsibility to individuals and family members, a shift also seen globally, where the benefits of family care over institutional care are increasingly emphasized (Lloyd, 2012). If institutional care is too costly, keeping people out of institutions seems, as Dalmer (2019) argues, intuitively the right solution, yet one that almost immediately created the cascading problem of a 'non-sustainable burden of care' for families (National Conference on Home Care, 1998). Yet the conceptualization of the purpose of home care has relentlessly shifted from a suite of services intended to support vulnerable people to live well at home to a cost-effective alternative to institutional care – that is to say, an obvious 'solution' to larger system issues (Ceci and Purkis, 2011). However, for home to be a solution, changes needed to be made in understanding what home care was 'for', to whom various responsibilities for care would belong, and how these responsibilities would be realized, with the 1990s marking the beginning of a significant reorganization in the ways health and support services were provided in home settings.

As alluded to in our Preface, at a time when changes were being implemented that altered responsibilities for care at home, the purposes and delivery of home care services were also changing in line with those policy changes. What is rendered all but invisible as policies shifted responsibilities for care are the ways that families were being drawn into everyday care at home in new ways, while, as Lloyd (2012, p 111) argues, policy-makers remained preoccupied with the overarching aim of cost containment. With cost containment identified as the most pressing problem, almost everyone was galvanized by mechanisms directed towards efficiency as such – in care at home these included technologies such as standardized assessment tools, performance indicators and outcome measures – alongside faith that attention to these sorts of processes would resolve most issues (Ceci and Purkis, 2011). These approaches and policies shifted the mix of formal and informal care, and prioritized the 'management' of needs through redefining and restricting eligibility for services, categorizing needs in ways that made them measurable by focusing on physical functioning, and attaching time and money to specific tasks as performance indicators (Björnsdóttir, 2009; Sim-Gould and Martin-Matthews, 2010; Ceci and Purkis, 2011, Lloyd, 2012).

For many decades now, any serious contribution to the discussion of support at home for older people, including those living with dementia, attends to institutionalized concerns for cost-effectiveness, efficiency and utility in relation to larger system issues, and, as Hollander notes, everything – funding, vision, practices – flows from how the purpose of home care, and care at home, is conceptualized (Hollander and Saskatchewan Health, 2006). That is to say, different purposes express differences in intention and emphasis that in turn shape how arguments are able to be expressed. In some senses the debate in the Canadian context since the 1990s has been shaped, and constrained, by this shift in discourse – if care at home is posed as a solution to a problem happening elsewhere in the system, that is, the economic viability of formal health and social care services, the discussion of just how home will be a 'solution' tends also to be rendered in that same economic vocabulary, leaving little space for consideration of the conditions and complexity of care or, in some cases, the enormity of the task that care at home may entail.

As we will discuss in Chapter 2, the discourses contained in most national dementia plans are similar in adopting the rationale of healthcare scarcity with dementia figured as a 'ticking time bomb', threatening to overwhelm limited resources. Similar as well is the embedded assumption that what care people living with dementia may need is best provided by, or is the responsibility of, unpaid family members who are 'supported', 'guided' and increasingly 'trained' to undertake this 'work' by state-provided health and social care services. Although the specific set of services to be offered families reflects each nation's historical social welfare structure, across nations, including Canada, dementia plans emphasize the need to support family carers, with critical support for these carers frequently highlighting a need for more education, training and counselling in order to help 'preserve their quality of life and resiliency and ... help sustain or increase their availability as caregivers' (CAHS, 2019, p xiii). Interestingly, a number of early analyses of the shift of care to home settings were rendered not only in terms of economic or cost-benefit analyses, but seemed compelled to try to grapple with the unquantifiable nature of care provision. As Parent and Anderson (1999, p 42) noted, 'there is no effective measure for determining appropriate levels of home support for individuals'. Although this could be read as a call for the development of better measures, Hollander and Chappell's (2001) more comprehensive study of the cost-effectiveness of home care underlines this problem of calculability. For example, they raise, but not surprisingly do not answer, the question of what level of burden is appropriate for family members. Indeed, it is not even entirely clear what kind of question this is. Undoubtedly in our current context Hollander and Chappell's sort of question persists, and is key in planning and providing home care services, but responding to it has remained a significant policy challenge.

Setting out the 'problem' in this way draws us to a place of urgency, showing the multiple ways dementia as such comes immediately to be entangled with social values and political economies, ideologies of individualism and family responsibility, slippages and ambiguities in negotiating public goods and private troubles. And it is certainly an urgency that mobilizes many diverse and worthy research and planning agendas concerned with finding a 'cure', improving 'care' or ensuring 'systems' will work efficiently and effectively when confronted with this problem. These efforts are significant, and their effects far reaching, and while we recognize the value of this work, in this book we explore a different track, one that runs alongside what could be described as the noisy and insistent clamouring for action. So while we acknowledge the louder discourses, it seems to us they already have many means of making themselves felt – institutions, experts and the full weight of Hacking's (2007) other engines of science and discovery cohere and converge in a crisis narrative that is familiar to almost everyone.

Our book, we could say, is a quieter book that, without denying the urgency and seriousness of what we are dealing with, tries to develop a different sense of the problem, to open some space to appreciate what Savransky (2018, p 217) describes as the 'thickness' of problems. Our research does not necessarily challenge the 'received wisdom and practice' so much as question the seeming clarity it offers (Cohen, 1998, p xvi), and, as noted earlier, by running alongside the more usual responses, adds some further dimensions to the situation in order that we may respond to it more fully.

The centrepiece of our writing is an ethnographic study of care at home when one family member has a diagnosis of dementia, and our experiences with this study, with the participant families and those involved with them are what have led us to try to formulate the problem of care at home in a somewhat different register. Ethnographic practice is often a space of disjuncture, challenging what we think we know about the world and how people live in it (McGranahan, 2014). And it is probably the outcome of any ethnographic practice to be unable to sustain 'a position' when experiences in a field produce interesting juxtapositions and challenges to dominant collective narratives. The collective representation of the 'crisis' of dementia certainly has felt presence in the everyday of our study, part of 'the social' through which dementia comes to matter for the families involved. But it is this latter point that forms the central question that organizes our writing, that is, what are the ways that dementia comes to matter in the everyday lives of families? What we have learned through the conduct of our research is in some ways simple, even obvious: every person 'does' dementia differently, and every family has to work out how, in their own singular and situated ways, to make things work. Formal systems try to help. Sometimes things work out, sometimes they don't, and often there is tension between home and system. The question for us, however, is how best to think about this situation – one that is well known and extensively studied – in a way that will help make it different, that will open it up to a transformation of some kind (Finlayson, 2006). That change is necessary is one part of the argument of this book; that change is possible is the other.

Both aspects of our argument rely on a philosophical practice of problematization, which, at its heart, is concerned with turning the given into a question (Foucault, 1989a; Rabinow, 2005). The objective, in Foucault's (1989b, pp 462–3) terms, is to 're-examine evidence and assumptions, to shake up habitual ways of working and thinking, to dissipate conventional familiarities, to re-evaluate rules and institutions' and from a 'reproblematization' contribute to the formation of something new. It seems possible in the case of care at home for people living with dementia, where research efforts have been massive, and outcomes often disappointing, that the nature of the problem we are dealing with still eludes us, or that efforts oriented to the acquisition of a certain number of 'facts' are not quite sufficient to help us meet the situation. All of which raises a question, as Finlayson (2006, p 542) argues, of 'how we turn the events and facts of the world into problems of various kinds', and, more specifically in our case here and now, how we have turned the ensemble of difficulties posed by cognitive changes associated with ageing into, as described earlier, a 'dementia epidemic' to be met by a shift of care to home settings, which, in turn, brings about a 'crisis in caring' at home.

Certainly it is possible to name some of the necessary associations – a particular political economy that de-emphasizes institutional care (Ulmanen and Szebehely, 2015), the increasing biomedicalization of ageing (Moreira and Palladino, 2008; Latimer, 2018), the dismantling of the social welfare state (Ong, 2006; Rose and Miller, 2010), the shift to market-driven governance (Simonet, 2008; Somers, 2008; Liveng, 2011), the devaluing of care work generally as well as policy approaches that highlight 'home is best' (Björnsdóttir, 2002), particularly when legitimated with reference to the 'unsustainable' care burden represented by older people (Ceci et al, 2012). These associations do not 'make' the problem of 'care at home', but they do contribute to its current sense. That is, as modes of social response, they contribute to how the sense of the problem is currently developed and expressed: what is to be *done* in the face of this 'dementia epidemic'? This question makes the 'problem' of growing old and experiencing cognitive changes visible in a particular way, one that seems to proceed directly to urgent forms of intervention intended to alleviate concerns associated with the costs of growing old.

It is this context that makes us want to pause, to slow down our thinking and doing, and, as Stengers (2005b, p 994) suggests, 'create an opportunity to arouse a slightly different awareness of the problems and situations mobilizing us'. If we start with the observation that many people living with dementia live at home with their families, it seems clear that much hangs on the question of how we understand this situation, including, but not limited to, the question of what may be done. It seems worth creating some space for hesitation, to recognize that the questions this situation holds do not merely reflect the limits of knowledge or our methods of knowing – to believe this is to believe that 'problems would go away if we simply knew more or differently' (Savransky, 2018, p 216). Rather, in the historical, that is to say, unfinished, unfolding of the world, events such as 'care at home' pose problems, but these are 'posed in the form, not of a prescription, but of a noisy, complicated question' (Savransky, 2018, p 218). Thus part of our intention with this book, through sharing the events of our research, is to contribute to elaborating a context where new questions are able to push through.

About the study

Our research began with the simple observation noted previously: many people living with dementia often live at home with their families. In the North American healthcare literature, the idea of families providing care to ailing family members, primarily older family members, has been discussed since the late 1940s. Over time, this recognition was transformed into the psychosocial concept of 'caregiver burden' and, from the 1970s to the present, it has been measured using increasingly complex techniques and calculations. While early research was motivated by an interest to 'relieve or reduce' the care burden (Zarit et al, 1980; Mohide et al, 1988), and to thus improve family carers' quality of life, 30 years later such ambitious aims were acknowledged to remain unmet (Zarit and Femia, 2008). Although it seems likely that some portion of the failure to adequately assist family carers will always be an outcome of local political conditions, our analysis (Purkis and Ceci, 2015) of the development and use of the concept of the 'care burden' in much dementia care research suggested that key assumptions defining the research field may contribute to its limited effectiveness. Using Alvesson and Sandberg's (2013) methodology of problematization, we surveyed 'care burden' research literature and reviews published between 1980 and 2012, and then closely analysed key texts to identify the presuppositions that were influencing research practices, including those that delineated the subject matter in question. Notably, in many of these studies we observed an almost exclusive focus on the isolated caregiver–recipient dyad as both object of inquiry and target of interventions, as well as an absence of an analysis of the materiality of care and caregiving practices.

Through this analysis (Purkis and Ceci, 2015) we came to see that although dominant methodologies have developed important knowledge about caregiving, they have also, through their successful efforts of dividing people up, worked to cleanse sites of caregiving of any evidence that there is anything beyond the individuals themselves involved in the actual practices of caregiving. That is to say, the whole gamut of practicalities, the multiplicity of material and organizational worlds that shape daily life – almost none of this was evident in the research literature. This, we argued, would have a significant impact on the knowledge produced and, given the high volume of research related to care burden and its acknowledged low impact, it seemed timely to rethink approaches to research and practice. It was on this basis that we developed and conducted the study described in this book.

Rather than the tightly bound triad of caregiver type, problem behaviour and tailored intervention found in traditional intervention studies, and the tendency to treat both caregiving and living with dementia as isolatable from other parts of life, we tried to approach the situation of caring for a family member living with dementia with a relational logic (Law, 1994, 2008; Mol et al, 2010; Moser, 2011; Pols, 2012) through which the elements of everyday life – people, objects, physical spaces, technologies and institutions – are understood to have significance and achieve their form and effects only in relation to one another. So rather than 'cleanse' caregiving situations of this multiplicity of elements, we tried to see how they were arranged and with what effects. The central point is that an approach that describes and accounts for the multiplicity of actors and arrangements – human, but also technological, physical and institutional – offers wider possibilities for action in terms of care (Moser, 2011). Our intention was to use these insights to develop a better understanding of what are 'good' or enabling arrangements for dementia care at home. In this we hoped to contribute to a growing body of dementia care literature that works to understand and account for the complex contexts of family caregiving (see, for example, de la Cuesta, 2005; Graham and Bassett, 2006; Askham et al, 2007; Moser, 2010; de la Cuesta-Benjumea, 2010; Gillies, 2012; Egdell, 2013; Berry, 2014).

Our study, *Delaying Institutionalization, Sustaining Families: Case Studies of Care at Home for People with Dementia*, was undertaken to learn more about how families are handling everyday life in the context of dementia, with the idea that if what families were already doing was better understood, their own efforts could be better supported. It is probably important to explain here how we are thinking about the term 'dementia'. The ongoing inability to define a cause or a cure for Alzheimer's disease, or to offer a definitive diagnosis except post mortem, has led to dementia associated with older age being seen less as an identifiable 'disease' and more as a 'recognizable cultural complex based on interpretations of normal, if problematic, biological and neurological variations in aging' (Gaines and Whitehouse, 2006, p 61; see also Gubrium, 1986; Holstein, 2000; Davis, 2004; Åsberg and Lum, 2010; Richards and Brayne, 2010; Lock, 2013; Portacolone et al, 2014). Gaines and Whitehouse (2006) also remind us that a critical issue related to dementia is the ability to carry out activities of daily life – dementia matters in terms of the ability to hold everyday life together and that ability is relative to context, resources and requirements – that is, what people are expected to do and what conditions are in place to help them. This perspective is key to our research as the issue we are most concerned with is how families handle a growing mismatch between the person living with dementia, the conduct of everyday life and fellow beings (Moser, 2008). Thus the specificities of diagnostic category, for example type or stage of dementia, are not foregrounded, but rather we are concerned with the practicalities of living with a dementia that has a range of effects.

Our focus was learning about the arrangements for care that are worked out by families in the course of their everyday circumstances. In this research the activities of families were understood as *care practices* to reflect the view that '*care* takes place in various shapes and forms' (Pols, 2012, p 17, emphasis in original), and that there are many activities beyond what is traditionally understood as caregiving that constitute care (see also Mol et al, 2010). For instance, in going along with a family to a doctor's visit, we learn about the practicalities of daily life that are troublesome, that are not necessarily 'about' dementia, but that still need to be 'cared for'– negotiating a walking frame across an uneven pavement, assessing the accessibility of a public toilet, managing the contingencies of bad weather or inconvenient and expensive parking. Or we see the practical understanding of 'how things work' embedded in a binder of information filled with community contacts and potential resources, organized into health, community, financial and legal sections. An artefact such as this binder embodies diverse assumptions – that there is indeed a world set up to respond to requests, that this world is divided in a predictable way, and that navigating this world effectively may be part of being a 'good' or responsible caregiver.

In our study of family care practices we tried to take account of this range of activities, actors and relations that help to sustain people's everyday lives. However, our attention is not focused on this form of complexity for its own sake, but rather for what we could learn of the networks of care that work to sustain people and relations, including social and material arrangements that enable the distribution of the work, care and risks of everyday living for people living with dementia and their families. Most simply, we were concerned with what makes it possible or impossible, easier or more difficult, to care for a family member living with dementia at home. The elements of everyday living are, by nature, heterogeneous, and our methodological and theoretical choices guided us to try to attend to these features rather than set them aside.

When everyday living becomes problematic for families, questions of how to carry on, how to adjust or adapt, frequently take centre stage, and as Collier and Lakoff (2005) suggest, being in the realm of the 'how to' always involves a certain idea of practices. We take the notion of care practices as a 'loose concept' (Ceci et al, 2017) in the sense that its content is not determined in advance but rather needs specifying empirically. In a general way, however, we looked to people's practices of handling daily life, adapting to specific circumstances and making things work from one day to the next (Mol et al, 2010). In some respects, care practices have an orientation to the 'good' but only to the extent that such practices aim at improving or stabilizing the situation of the people or things cared for – but this, too, needs specification in actual situations. The notion of a care practice is also 'loose' because it is possible to trace elements to different places with which they have relations. The sociality of practices is given from the outset; to be in a practice means to actively and knowledgeably engage an environment constituted in and by people, relations, materialities and discourses (Palsson, 1994).

We recognize that some ambiguity lies in the language of 'care practices', and there is the possibility of confusing or conflating family care practices and the professional care practices of doctors, nurses or other formal helpers. However, families and formal carers are engaged in quite different ways in care at home, and we will argue throughout the book that understanding these as distinct practices of care, with distinct requirements and obligations, is part of how we might work to better support families. To meet families as the protagonists of their own stories seems to require, at the very least, recognition of their knowledgeable and ongoing practical accomplishments as they engage, as Stengers (2018, p 149) might say, in a practice of 'worlding the world, of having the world matter'.

How to write about this is a question – one way we think about this, and try to show it, is to challenge those ways of thinking that locate dementia 'in' the person so diagnosed, and to show that dementia, where it is a problem, is actually a problem 'in' family practices and arrangements, that dementia is something found in interactions and daily life (Moser, 2010). In every case and in every story, the family member living with dementia is both actively present and actively contributing to the family care practices – we observed no family member as 'merely' a passive recipient of others' actions. One aspect of writing that makes this reality less visible is the way that the verbal comes to be privileged – both in society and at times in the telling of our stories – as carrying the means of agency and action. In the writing of the stories, we did try to show each actor as part of and as having an effect on the arrangements – for example, a family outing that shows how all actors are in relation, responsive to each other and essential to accomplishing the activity. We describe such a situation in Chapter 5.

In many of our descriptions we also try to show people are present and active, influencing the progress of everyday events, resistant to some things, acquiescent to others. That is to say, we try to show, as Schillmeier (2017, p 56) has observed, 'care is not generally divided between the carers and the cared for, but distributed among the different actors involved'. But it was also the case that among our participant families, the person carrying the dementia diagnosis was not very verbal – except for Albert,[1] each had different communicative challenges that we may not have been entirely successful in representing. So this may be both a limitation of the written form and our ability to fully convey the ways non-verbal conduct is influencing the action.

The book

As noted previously, the centrepiece of our writing is an ethnographic study of care at home when one family member has a diagnosis of dementia. Data collection for the study was undertaken in two midsize Western Canadian cities between 2014 and 2019. To learn about family care practices, the practicalities they handle and their relations with multiple social and material contexts, we used traditional ethnographic methods of observation, interview and document analysis (Hammersley and Atkinson 2007). Ethnographic methods allowed us to go and see people and objects 'in action', and to participate, where possible, in the practices of families. The fieldwork with families took place from 2015 to 2017, and during this time four families were followed by the first author (Christine Ceci) for periods of four months to one year, beginning with their enrolment in the study and ending when circumstances had become such that the institutionalization of their family member was decided on. 'Following' a family meant going along with members of a family on visits to doctors' offices, day programmes, caregiver support groups and social outings, as well as visiting their homes for informal conversation or to be present during visits from various healthcare providers.

Detailed overviews of each family's story and involvement with the study are presented in Chapter 4. For each family we offer a descriptive case history, drawing extensively on our Field notes to highlight key aspects of their experiences of living with dementia. Our case examples are intended to be illustrative and instructive rather than representative of something larger (Mol and Law, 2002), a means to sensitize us to the issues and complexities of families negotiating everyday life with dementia. The information shared in this chapter provides us with material to think with, and sets the stage for reading the chapters that follow (Chapters 5–8).

However, before turning to the family stories, we offer two chapters that describe aspects of the study that occurred outside of the main fieldwork and that help to explain how we came to analyse the family stories in the way that we did. Prior to our fieldwork with families, we conducted interviews with 14 key informants active in the local context of dementia care in order to learn about the context families were dealing with from the perspectives of those occupying formal roles intended to help individuals diagnosed with a dementia and their family members. In selecting our sample, we were not looking for an exhaustive number of individuals to interview but rather one or two from each organizational 'level' representing agencies and members of healthcare teams in the community who speak to and advise family members on options for accessing community-based support. In interviews, we asked the informants to talk about their primary responsibilities related to the care of individuals with a diagnosis of dementia living in the community. We asked about the major issues they see families facing, about gaps in support for individuals and families, and what plans they were aware of to respond to those gaps. In this way we were seeking to develop a descriptive analysis of the work of planning dementia care strategies at a population level, and how that compares with the actual work of helping individuals and families.

In Chapter 2 we analyse the accounts of these key informants – those responsible for planning programmes of support for people with dementia as well as those who had responsibility for implementing those programmes as they engaged in work to draw rather abstract strategies down into everyday life. Through this analysis we begin to understand the ways the discourses of a 'dementia epidemic' have worked to both overdetermine and underdefine the problems of individuals and families living with a dementia. As an overdetermined problem, the coming 'crisis' demands the attention of those who occupy positions of responsibility for financing and planning formal health services as well as those in positions to develop community-based responses to support those ageing in the community. The metaphor of a 'rising tide' (Dudgeon, 2010) or 'grey tsunami' has come to stand for the sense of dread that health service administrators, politicians, healthcare workers and many members of the public live under as they live their increasingly busy lives, facing increasing numbers of urgent priorities. As an underdefined problem, the 'grey tsunami' represents the conceptual space generated by population statistics indicating that people are living longer, developing more chronic illnesses as they age, while at the same time birth rates are declining, resulting in a bottom-line calculation of larger numbers of older people with fewer younger people available to care and support them. And it greatly underdefines the actual problems of such a changing population distribution: each older person, each family, is unique and so each needs something different than the next. The tensions we observed here speak to Gronemeyer's (2017, p 20) observation that a major issue for society is the many ways that 'dementia evades planning'.

In Chapter 3 we continue to think about the differences in terms of what is at stake for those involved in different ways in the 'problem' of care at home. We suggest that tensions among the 'interests' of those involved – people living with dementia and their families, service providers and policy-makers – remain undertheorized. To access and understand some of these different ways of thinking we made a film from our ethnographic data, and then used this film as a starting point for discussion among these differently positioned groups. Analysis of participants' responses to the film suggested to us that although families, providers and policy-makers are related through common interests, they do not necessarily have the same interests in common. We do not argue that these diverging interests are a problem. Instead, we draw on Stengers' (2005a, 2005b, 2015 [2009], 2019) ecology of practices to suggest that rather than seeking an alignment of interests around one or another 'best' practice, working for the creation of moments of rapport when 'something' good may be done in the 'here and now' is a more pragmatic and humane move.

Our experiences with these discussion groups were pivotal to our thinking about the nature of family care practices, raising the persistent question of what are good ways to think about how family care practices and those of the formal system relate. This is, of course, not a new question. There is a vast literature extending over many decades exploring questions of the relations between informal and formal carers, alongside many different frameworks for conceptualizing these relations (see, for example, Twigg, 1989; Bond, 1992; Lyons and Zarit, 1999; Zarit et al, 1999; Ward-Griffin and McKeever, 2000; Wiles, 2003; Büscher et al, 2011; Stephan et al, 2018; O'Shea et al, 2019). Yet despite significant research, Lyons and Zarit's early observation that we are unlikely to find a 'perfect interface' (1999, p 191) seems still to be the case. Explanations of the difficulties in the encounter are also diverse, highlighting the complexities of the relations involved, the absence of a shared perspective on what needs to be done, differing value systems, as well as the need to locate issues arising in the specific contexts of care. While relations between formal and informal carers are by no means always found to be adversarial (Carpentier and Grenier, 2012), there are persistent difficulties including that families may find accessing formal services more burdensome than caregiving itself (Stephan et al, 2018), or that they receive only ambiguous benefit from doing so (Lloyd and Stirling, 2011). Specific kinds of supportive services such as respite, which may be potentially helpful to families, are also found not to do as much good as is hoped for (Stirling et al, 2014; O'Shea et al, 2017). So, despite extensive research and practice efforts, the issue of uneasy relations persists.

Elaborating good ways to think about how family care practices and those of the formal system relate is a longstanding theoretical and practical problem. In Chapter 5 we delve more deeply into Isabelle Stengers' (2005a, 2005b, 2015 [2009], 2019) thinking about an 'ecology of practices' to theorize divergences in family and formal care practices that have implications for care. In Stengers' view, what makes a practice diverge is also what makes it a particular practice; overriding these differences and imposing similarity, such as efforts to 'professionalize' family caregiving, can damage the practice so aligned. Instead, Stengers' figure of the diplomat shows how diverging practices that have common interests – but not necessarily the same interests – might relate. Examples from our study show the relevance of this ecological theorizing of differences and the need for diplomatic relations between practices that leave 'borders' and thus practices intact.

Chapter 6 builds from the specificities of family care practices described in Chapters 4 and 5 to consider the difficulties in keeping and caring for family practices. We start from the observation that dealing biomedically with dementia brings with it a set of activities that work to name and frame dementia, significant because once named and framed, the reality of dementia becomes patterned, and once patterned, in turn, patterns what is being done. To see this patterning we examine the processes by which dementia has come to matter for the families involved in the research – the practices through which dementia is experienced, named, measured, treated and drawn into other social discourses, practices that not only tell about what dementia currently 'is', but also the social moment we are in (Cohen, 1998).

This questioning does not suggest that there is no 'real' dementia or problematic situations to be dealt with, but simply that there is also a patterning of dementia that is a product of local and contingent practices. Questions of patterning can be highlighted or left in the background – but if highlighted, they generate a complexity in understanding family experiences of dementia that can't be flattened out. It is this complexity that is the focus of this chapter. How do assumptions about the nature of the problem contribute to the ongoing shape of care? We will argue that moving beyond a predominantly biomedical framework starts with recognition of the multiplicity of enactments of dementia, and of specificities of care related to time and place – that is, how life is shaped and negotiated on an ongoing basis.

In Chapter 7 we revisit Gronemeyer's (2017, p 20) assertion that 'dementia evades planning' by exploring the borders of helpfulness through our case studies, particularly the question of whether health and social care systems, at least in their current configurations, can do more than 'prop up' families. What would sustaining families look like? In previous chapters we map out the rough outlines of the system through families' experiences: how people deal with what they find problematic. And then, when they need help, what helpfulness looks like and what our stories show us about how help could be fostered with both family members as well as formal care providers, empowered to contribute to accomplishing helpful relations. Recognizing that helpfulness cannot be predetermined challenges and has implications for policy and planning services. The previous chapters show different matters of concern among those differently positioned in relation to care at home, and the case studies reinforce the issue of divergence by showing that family care practices differ significantly from those of system actors – together, these analyses support an argument against single solution approaches.

Our closing chapter reflects on our argument as a whole. The challenges families living with a diagnosis of dementia experience show how care in the community is currently thought, and also that there are gaps in our thinking about the nature of 'care' in this setting. What 'kind' of community is demanded by a problem like dementia, a problem that often seems to evade our best efforts at planning (Gronemeyer, 2017)? One limitation, we argue, lies in our framing of care, and we make a case for a turn from individualized, individualizing notions of care. Instead, we try to think of the implications of attending to care as diverse arrangements made up of people, things, institutions, discourses, normativities, knowledges and the relations made among all of these. Different assumptions are built into different arrangements, including what the diagnosis is and is not, whose problem it is and is not, or where the problem is located, for example, the idea that dementia is something located in people's minds. This seems to us significant, especially in light of Mol's (2002) argument that different arrangements create different enactments of disease. The looser thinking of arrangements allows us to think different thoughts, for instance, what kind of 'dementia' do we want to have? What is actually possible?

Developing a different sense of the problem

Earlier we made the statement that this is a quieter book, at least quieter than the loud and urgent calls for action that many of us have become accustomed to (and accustomed to making). Contrary to what is often found in policy texts, this book does not answer the question, what is to be *done* in the face of this so-called dementia epidemic? Rather, we pose some key questions for those who make policy as well as those who practice in the spaces created by policy, and in so doing illustrate why, as noted earlier, we have chosen to write a quieter book that we hope interrupts the clarity of settled plans and adds new dimensions to the situation. So, rather than asking what is to be done, we paraphrase Stengers (2015 [2009], p 88), and ask instead, what does trying to respond to 'dementia' 'in a way that isn't barbaric call for?' 'Barbaric' is a harsh and unsettling word, but it references something important. Around this 'problem' of dementia many different groups are gathered with many different interests and concerns, as well as different ways of presuming to already know what the situation demands – and from whom. In some sense all these differences make the situation what it currently is – they contribute to the ways a common concern is able to emerge. The clamour alerts us to the seriousness of things, but also has the possibility of freezing the landscape. It is this location, where certainty about what can be done struggles with its limits, that Stenger's (2007) words cited at the outset of the chapter have both resonance and relevance. They tell us not what is to be done, but *how* we might approach the problems with which we are concerned: 'Making a situation, past or present, be of importance, means intensifying the sense of possibles it harbours, as expressed by the struggles and claims to another way of making it exist' (p 7). The work of our book leans towards this speculative impulse in the sense of rejecting or resisting what Stengers (2007) describes as the 'lure of purification' (p 2), a move necessary if we are to enable different possibilities to emerge. 'To exclude nothing,' writes Stengers, 'means resisting the terms of the alternatives that so inexorably seem to foist themselves upon us, leading to false choices' (p 3).

In this situation, a situation whose 'already knowns' seem so difficult to resist, we use our data, the families' stories and those of others we talked with, to think with, and to develop possibly helpful ideas and ways of framing the situation – and in attempting to present the situation a little differently, intervening in it (Stengers, 2015 [2009]). But not in the sense of 'unveiling' the truth of things, or, as Stengers writes, making claims that would allow us to 'pass from perplexity to knowledge' (2015 [2009], p 34). Rather, in loosening things up a little we try to add some relevant dimensions but without accruing to ourselves the power to define the situation, to say 'this' is what is really going on (Savransky and Stengers, 2018). The point, really, is to give the situation itself – care at home for people living with a dementia – the power to make us ask more varied and interesting questions, questions that might eventually change the conditions for engaging with it. It is to make that Foucauldian kind of effort: 'from the moment one begins to be unable, any longer, to think things as one usually thinks them, transformation becomes simultaneously very urgent, very difficult, and altogether possible' (Foucault, 1982a, p 34).

Note

[1]   Pseudonyms have been used for all participants to protect anonymity.

2

From strategy to service: practices of identification and the work of organizing dementia services

Sociomaterial associations and a 'looming catastrophe'

In Chapter 1 we explained how we intend to examine the ways in which families make arrangements in life when they are caring for a family member with a diagnosis of dementia. We described our approach as one informed by a relational logic where elements of everyday life take their form and effects only in relation to one another (Law, 1994, 2008; Mol et al, 2010; Moser, 2011; Pols, 2012). Approaching the topic of dementia from a relational stance means that we examine what Law and Mol (1995, p 274) describe as 'associations'. Law and Mol do not limit the availability of associations just to human actors; they advance the possibility that 'association is a matter not only for social beings, but also one to do with materials' (1995, p 274). This means that in this chapter we can broaden our gaze somewhat to examine the context within which families arrange care for their family member diagnosed with dementia. And we can include people, offices, websites, documentation, national plans and even ideas that are operating with a relational logic that makes up dementia care within the location where our study was conducted.

So, while our interest throughout this research project has been on the families and their practices of caring for one of their family members diagnosed with dementia, we also knew from the beginning that formal health services operating from hospitals, clinics, medical offices and community health centres would play some part in those care practices. And these formal services themselves, as well as families so affected, are associated with those discursive associations setting out what dementia 'is' and what should, on a population scale, be done about it.

We begin this chapter with an examination of some key historical developments relevant to the work of those who are responsible for planning and providing health and social service support for people living with dementia. We examine those historical developments as materials available to such planners enabling particular ways of organizing social beings – themselves as well as the people living with dementia and their family support. This question of associations and what they produce is critical to our analysis of that work.

Following this discussion we provide an overview of the key informant interviews that were part of our study, including a section that sets out our method for analysing those interviews. Then we introduce the conceptual framework offered by Law and Mol (1995) that assists us in telling a story of how dementia support services were operating at the time of our research. Our interest is in showing how social beings and materials operate in a relational logic such that they build associations aimed at stabilizing big, complex problems like dementia. Our interviews with key informants offer ample evidence of the sort of ideas and strategies they have developed that help them in this work. And they also offer some evidence of the limits of the strategy. This is also very important because, in later chapters, when we focus more on the families themselves, we see and hear about their struggles – about how they seek support and how often that support does not quite provide the sort of help they were hoping for. If we are to understand the struggles of families, these limits in the extent to which plans actually provide help are important to understand.

From private troubles to political strategy

The history of dementia is one marked by quite radical revisions in societal understanding of ageing and cognitive decline. As Ballenger (2017, p 713) notes,

> everything we know about the natural history of age-associated progressive dementia suggests that it has always been part of human experience, but only since the early twentieth century has dementia been regarded as the product of a disease, and only in the last half of the twentieth century has it been regarded as a major public health issue. This broad reframing of dementia was the result not merely of changing medical concepts but of a broader social transformation of aging.

Ballenger points to one of the key transition points occurring in the early 20th century when the understanding of cognitive decline in older adults changed from being simply a feature expected as part of normal ageing into a specific disease process – and importantly, one for which treatments and even a cure might be found. Further, he raises a second key transformation, that of dementia now understood as a disease more widely prevalent in the population than previously thought. In this way, dementia has become a disease process of such magnitude that its designation as a 'major public health issue' was established and advanced for further actions.

Neither of these major redefinitions of dementia occurred without significant debate among interested communities. Beard (2016) offers some interesting insights here. She notes the appearance of increasingly more specific sub-forms of dementia. These were created under the broader diagnosis of Alzheimer's disease and included behavioural observations that, at the time of death, could be associated with changes in brain structure. The first of these precursors to Alzheimer's disease was mild cognitive impairment (MCI), and later, with an increasing focus on early diagnosis, a precursor to MCI, prodromal subjective cognitive impairment (SCI). These new diagnoses emerged during significant debate within the neurological community, especially as members tried to determine if MCI could be considered a separate form of dementia or whether it was a precursor to Alzheimer's disease:

> Although MCI as a separate nosological entity allegedly allows 'active rather than palliative care', the demarcation between normal aging and disease remains vague and the legal implications of conceptualizing memory loss as abnormal is equally Byzantine. Due to these factors, many vociferously argued that consensus on the criteria of diagnosing MCI needed to include not only clinicians and researchers in the field, but individuals studying bioethics, legal specialists, and those concerned with classification systems. Unfortunately, these pleas were not heeded when the proposal for changing the diagnostic criteria for AD [Alzheimer's disease] lengthened the disease process even further … (extending) the medical gaze to include two new phases prior to Alzheimer's: prodromal subjective cognitive impairment (SCI) and MCI. (Beard, 2016, pp 33–4)

Interestingly, Beard (2016) notes that while experts closed ranks at this earlier stage of diagnostic category development, later the need to increase access to a population of people on whom to test emerging diagnostic categories as well as experimental pharmaceutical treatments created a very particular role for patient involvement. Beard points to a double-edged sword faced by older people eager join others with 'similar biological abnormalities to coalesce in the promotion of research into the cause and cure of their specific conditions' (2016, p 39). This association between older adults worried about early and pathological cognitive impairment and scientists interested in advancing knowledge on a topic of broad societal import 'is simultaneously a potential tool for empowerment and a device of regulation' (Beard, 2016, p 39). As a tool for empowerment, this association between patients and their families alongside medical scientists and neurologists interested in advancing the science of dementia and developing a range of potential pharmaceutical interventions to address some of the serious impacts of dementia has indeed been powerful. Together they have contributed to lifting dementia up from its location in the family home as a set of quite private troubles and into the more public domain where it has certainly, as Ballenger (2017) noted, become a public health issue. In this context, we begin to see the associations developing further and now being constituted by people living with dementia, their family members, scientists, public health personnel and advocacy organizations such as the Alzheimer's Association, banding together to place pressure on public officials to develop national strategies to address this problem. To the extent they are successful in this regard, we can, following Law and Mol (1995), say that these associations between older people worried about their memories, demographic trends and calculations, scientists, pharmaceutical companies and public health officials have been successful in their sociomaterial productivity to create something with sufficient stability as to be able to make itself a matter of concern for national governments.

Taking dementia seriously: national dementia strategy documents

In 2008, France became the first country to present a formal strategy to address growing concerns with increasing numbers of its citizens being diagnosed with dementia (Alzheimer Europe, nd). Their strategy was focused on three key activities: improve diagnosis, improve treatment and support services, and promote research. Since 2008, more than 30 nations have followed France's lead to develop their own national strategy to address dementia, framed as being a significant health concern affecting not only the person diagnosed with the disease, but also their family and the communities they live in (Chow et al, 2018). Canada has been among the last to develop and publicize its national strategy document. Published in 2019, *A Dementia Strategy for Canada: Together We Aspire*, offers three national objectives: prevent dementia, advance therapies and find a cure, and improve the quality of life of people living with dementia and caregivers (PHAC, 2019).

Framed a little differently, these three objectives are remarkably well aligned with the three key activities outlined 11 years previously by France.

Writing just ahead of the release of the Canadian strategy paper, Chow and her colleagues (2018) published a review paper in which they examined 25 existing national strategy documents. Their review indicated 'five major priorities' (2018, p 205) covered by most of these documents: increasing awareness of the disease, establishing support services, improving the standard of care, improving training and education for healthcare practitioners, and promoting research. Again, a remarkably strong alignment in terms of priority actions is evident in this analysis.

It seems at least plausible to draw the conclusion that the debates about whether dementia was simply a part of normal ageing versus a disease state have been settled, and the outcome, that it is a disease state, has been incorporated into these governmental documents. Similarly, the encouragement for funding to be directed towards research that might develop a cure for this disease also suggests an association with earlier efforts when the status of an Alzheimer's-type dementia was less settled. Now there are no debates. Dementia is a disease of sufficient concern that it warrants national attention and legitimacy as something that all citizens should be on the watch for – indeed, should have themselves tested for early so that participation in research and access to treatments might begin as early as possible. These priorities have associations with the earlier debates about the disease.

Less apparent in the early debates about dementia are interests associated with the priorities identified in the national plans related to standards of care, training of professional caregivers and the establishment of support services. These concerns appear to be linked in a quite specific way with what Ballenger argues was the reframing of dementia in the latter half of the 20th century from being simply an interesting disease to it becoming a 'major public health issue' (2017, p 713). Incorporated into these national plans is a recognition that people living with dementia will require care of a high standard and of a significant quantity. The national plans offer an indication at least that governments have an awareness that funding may need to be targeted to dementia as a public health concern – and it seems reasonable to assume that the reference to 'support services' would include support for care to be conducted in homes by families who would themselves require support.

Framed in this way, national strategy documents that take account of jurisdictionally relevant population characteristics are now possible.

Law and Mol (1995, p 274) note that 'when we look at the social, we are also looking at the production of materiality. And when we look at materials, we are witnessing the production of the social'. We advance the argument here that the debates that took place over the course of the 20th century can be understood in these terms: brain cells examined under microscopes making tangles and plaques visible produce patients diagnosed with dementia. Patients and their families, having participated in raising the profile of this new disease, and perhaps helping to frame it as demanding more care from families than what they can reasonably be expected to provide, produce national plans signalling priorities for government funding as well as philanthropic goals.

These historical associations undergird the context of work, offering categories for use by our key informants as they work to identify people living with dementia in the community in need of support. The associations further equip the key informants with strategic goals from which accounts are developed suggesting that, what a journalist in a major national newspaper refers to as the 'looming catastrophe' (Yang, 2015) of dementia, is instead a problem being actively worked on. Those accounts can then feature in responses suggesting resources are being put in place that will better prepare local communities for what is expected to come. These key informants, some of them in powerful senior leadership roles, direct efforts that seek to make a positive impact on the 'looming crisis' of dementia. They participate in the creation and then the distribution of strategies and processes that, through associations with social actors and materials, 'exert power' (Latour, 1984), organizing particular responses to the problem of dementia. We are interested in these relays of power, their operations and effects.

In the next section we discuss the methods used to obtain accounts of such work from key informants engaged in the work of planning for the 'looming crisis' and those who work directly with people diagnosed with dementia as they deal with the day-to-day concerns of living with that disease in the community. Following this, we delve into the accounts to examine how signs and strategies are employed by our key informants as they endeavour to stabilize (Law and Mol, 1995) the dementia problem.

Interviewing key informants

In order to understand how healthcare leaders looked at dementia – how it figured for them in their day-to-day work – we sought interviews with specific people, key informants, who worked in formal roles in health service planning and care delivery in the jurisdictions within which the ethnographic study was conducted – two urban centres in Western Canada. We spoke with people responsible for planning regional services for large metropolitan areas as well as more rural settings to a population of more than four million people. We spoke with people managing community-based health centres where programmes for people living with dementia are offered. We spoke with clinicians who visit people with a diagnosis of dementia in their homes. Our sampling strategy here was not to try to obtain a representative sample of health services workers. Rather, we were interested in speaking with people occupying different organizational locations where we thought interests, knowledge of effective care and perspectives would be different. We did not assume one location would have a better perspective than others – instead, we were interested in better understanding the characteristics of the relationships between the different locations.

In our conversations with our informants, we asked them to talk about their primary responsibilities related to the care of individuals with a diagnosis of dementia living in the community, about the major issues they see families facing as they work to care for their family member at home, and about gaps in the support of individuals and families and what plans they were aware of to respond to those gaps. Our analysis of the accounts offered by our key informants draws from an interpretive tradition where verbatim transcripts undergo close reading in order to develop empirical arguments about understandings of the world conveyed through speech. The approach takes as a starting point that our identities, whether as members of a family or members of a healthcare team, are much less settled than what we, in everyday conversation, assume is the case (Purkis, 2003, p 42). The American anthropologist, James Fernandez (1986, p vii), describes this approach as one that takes the person to be:

> a very generalized animal with very little in specific adaptations to specific milieus wired into our brains. As a consequence we are required to invent ways of being – from rules and plans to worldviews and cosmologies – more or less appropriate to any of the diverse milieus in which we have installed ourselves.

In the ordinary course of a workday, our key informants proceed in their activities as though their identities are settled. Rarely are they asked why they are approaching a situation in a particular way. Instead, and without being explicitly aware of it, they are operating on what, collectively, they and their team members have devised as being 'more or less appropriate' to their work contexts. In doing so, they draw on 'rules and plans' (Fernandez, 1986, p vii) that are collectively agreed on as relevant to the tasks they have been asked to achieve.

When we invited people to take part in interviews, our opportunity was to ask them questions that had the effect of unsettling their identity just a little, because we were asking them to develop an account of their understanding of how things work and why they engaged in the activities they did on a daily basis. These questions generated accounts more detailed than would be typical in explaining their everyday work practice. We sought from them their usual, practised account of themselves and their work – what Giddens (1984, p 41) refers to as an account derived from the discursive consciousness. When more detailed questions were asked of key informants in order to gain a deeper understanding of their practices, we approached those accounts as relying more heavily on what Giddens describes as their practical consciousness (1984, p 41). Giddens posits that informants engage in reflexive monitoring of their actions (including speech acts) and the settings in which those actions occur. Informants make readings of those settings and organizational contexts to draw up accounts of their practices that they believe will provide an accountable explanation of their actions for interviewers such as ourselves. The knowledgeability that an informant brings to a situation in order to create an account is rendered into the verbatim transcript, and serves as evidence of both discursive and practical consciousness.

In making a close reading of the transcripts, we looked for common explanations across accounts because these offered us an insight into those features of the organizational context that Giddens (1984, p 16) refers to as 'structures' or understandings through which social actions (such as the development of community-based programming to support people living in the community with a diagnosis of dementia) are achieved. At the same time, we sought out divergent explanations because these suggest that, in different locales and under different circumstances, different knowledge is necessary to describe the social world inhabited by organizational actors, and the family members and people living with dementia that they seek to assist.

Our analysis of the transcripts generated from our conversations with key informants, conducted on the basis of the philosophical position laid out here, illustrates activities in two distinct settings: first, activities taking place in offices and meeting rooms where jurisdictional plans to address dementia-as-an-organizational-problem are discussed and developed; and second, we analysed data derived from key informants who visited clients in their homes and in community-based agencies where people seek help with dementia-as-lived at home with a family member exhibiting signs of changing cognitive ability. Our aim in approaching our interviews and our analysis of those interviews in this way was to begin to excavate from the actual work of people faced with the challenges of dementia, as laid out in the national plans, some of those practical solutions that we had detected were missing from the wider literature on this topic. That is, if, as we suggested in Chapter 1, 'dementia' as such exists in a discursive space characterized by an overdetermination of incidence of dementia and an underdefinition of the means to respond effectively, what patterns of practice enable acts of translation between and within these locations. We draw on segments from our transcripts to illustrate how these key informants practise in this space and ultimately, how they utilize practices of identification to do this work.

A framework for studying relational logics

Law and Mol (1995) offer a conceptual framework that we will use to analyse what we see happening in our key informants' descriptions of their everyday practice as well as the organizational goals and strategies they identify and pursue in that work. In setting out the framework here, we include some examples from our interviews with key informants. These will be elaborated on in the longer narrative of the work of key informants that follows.

The first element of Law and Mol's (1995, p 275) framework is semiotics, by which they mean to point to the ways in which materials are relational effects. Further, they argue that social stability is linked to material distinction. For example, when we spoke with key informants, they talked with us about one of the key issues that they see facing families, which is the problem of navigation. We can think about navigation as an example of a semiotic relation. It suggests social relationships: someone coming alongside another to guide them along a complicated pathway. In the context of dementia, navigation suggests professional caregivers within the community gently guiding people with cognitive impairment from place to place. This is, in part, what our key informants told us was their goal – to set up a system in which, when people obtain a diagnosis of dementia, they would be linked into the health and social service system in such a way that they would know when and where to look for help and when to transition from one level of help to another. In this way navigation aims at stabilizing what is otherwise evidently a rather chaotic environment for people living with dementia. Navigation, in Law and Mol's terms, *performs* material distinctions – a community map of sorts that families would be able to tap into to answer their questions about where and when to seek help.

The second element of Law and Mol's (1995, p 275) framework is strategy. Strategy is also a matter of material distinction. Strategy suggests recursive and reflexive material distinction. Instead of helping us excavate examples of stability, however, strategy is all about social change. Once an idea like navigation has been surfaced as a problem for families and people living with dementia, programmes can then be designed that enable navigation. In our discussions with key informants, we were told about what we have come to think of as the 'ideal programme' for people with a dementia diagnosis. This involves a person seeking out an early diagnosis of dementia as day-to-day activities are experienced as problematic – perhaps the person finds it increasingly difficult to remember the names of familiar people or they forget they have promised to visit a friend and go to the grocery store instead. Such problems may indicate some cognitive impairment – or they might not. A visit to the doctor's office might help to determine which it is. Once there, and with a diagnosis made, the doctor's office then links the person with the community agency that has developed the ideal programme. The person then receives a follow-up visit every six months to monitor changes in cognitive functioning.

As an example of strategy, we can see such an ideal programme aiming to effect social change. Rather than people struggling to find support for their family member who is struggling with cognitive decline, the ideal programme will regularize their involvement with a community support organization and support will be initiated in a more proactive way. Law and Mol (1995) argue that strategy is a metaphor for thinking about the organization of materiality.

The final element of the framework is patchwork. Patchwork depends on a sensitivity to difference in the here and now. It depends on the possibility that social and material relations do not add up or hang together as a whole. Instead, the idea of patchwork means that, rather than being stable and capable of achieving social change, the relations between people and things are like a patchwork. What we thought were stabilities are unstable. Where we saw direction, we now see 'shakes and quivers' (Law and Mol, 1995, p 275). An example that we will explore a little later is one in which a programme director tells of a man who was simply driving by her office one day. He stops in to ask about resources for his wife who he thinks may have dementia. This programme director tells us that the ideal programme is great – but she encounters many people like this man. Rather than seeking out an early diagnosis from the family doctor and becoming part of the ideal programme, diagnosis is not sought until much later in the progression of the disease. As evidence of the instability of the programme that has been set up to enable navigation through a diagnosis and support for dementia, the programme director invites the man and his wife inside, and tells them not to worry – "we'll make it work".

The question we are left with regarding patchwork is this: is patchwork evidence of system failure? Or is it, perhaps, something of an inclusive failsafe when conditions permit its operation? This is a question we will return to at the end of this chapter.

The sociopolitical context of dementia

Before digging into the stories told to us by our key informants, we want to illustrate further contextual factors at play in the everyday work of anyone engaged in practices related to dementia. We raise these here because many of these influences are at play in a wider multinational context, and are rarely pointed to by people working in the sorts of work environments where we found our key informants. Indeed, they may not be directly aware of some of these influences. We raise them here because we can see traces of them, particularly in the strategies that our key informants spend so much energy on developing and sustaining through their relationships with other organizational actors as well as families and people living with dementia themselves. One of the most pressing priorities advanced by these multinational forces, one which we have previously noted is also present in every nation's 'dementia strategy', is the priority for 'increasing rates of diagnosis of dementia and cognitive impairment' (Le Couteur et al, 2013, p 1). The most frequent reason offered for the value of such a priority is that it affords health professionals time to offer counselling for advanced care directives, and it permits patients and families time to organize financial and future guardianship arrangements before the diagnosed person is incapable of making decisions that will be deemed legally competent (Le Couteur et al, 2013, p 3).

This same policy direction is advocated by regional and national health ministries and disease advocacy groups, and forms a central pillar, as noted previously, in the over 30 national dementia plans in existence today (Chow et al, 2018). Despite the effective spread of this policy directive, research exploring the effectiveness of early diagnosis as a benefit to patients and families suggests limited, if any, benefit (Waldorff et al, 2012; Le Couteur et al, 2013; Clarkson et al, 2012). Instead, the more critical view of this policy directive is that it primarily benefits pharmaceutical and biomedical companies in search of drug and, more recently, genetic treatments for dementia. Perhaps even more problematically is the fact that this policy directive aimed at early diagnosis is now deeply established in health and medical practices, even though, as Ballenger (2017, p 717) notes, owing to numerous recent failures of drug trials to demonstrate the benefits of pharmaceutical treatments, critics have begun to 'question whether (pharmaceutical) research is pursuing a dead end'. Added to this, Ballenger further notes the perhaps more important finding that 'the rate of dementia in the United States declined from 11.6 per cent to 8.8 per cent between 2000 and 2012' (2017, p 717), findings that contradict catastrophic stories that pepper social media and potentially undermine powerful financial partnerships operating between the pharmaceutical industry and disease lobby groups (Norton et al, 2013; Wu et al, 2016; Le Couteur et al, 2013).

Recognizing the powerful sway such influences have on the definition and relevance of any number of major disease categories, our goal in our own analysis is to try not to fall prey to any particular view of dementia in this chapter. Rather, our aim is to examine taken-for-granted ideas such as the one about the widely accepted value of early diagnosis as an example of a strategy in Law and Mol's (1995) terms – a material distinction that both performs and derives from semiotic stabilities to produce social change. And then, in the patchwork that is everyday practice, to be alert for evidence that could show how dementia, despite all its powerful influences and influencers, is not a settled matter. This is important because it is precisely how these stabilities and instabilities affect the families at the core of our work that will be addressed in later chapters.

Narratives of navigating a 'looming catastrophe'

Despite the controversies pointed to in the preceding sections, our key informants offered only occasional glimpses that dementia is anything other than a stable object and of significant social concern. As we transition here into our analysis of accounts provided by key informants, we begin with the following account because in it our informant provides a description of what we have called earlier the ideal programme.

The ideal programme

Our informant, a programme coordinator, lives in a medium-sized city and, in addition to providing services related to the ideal programme in town, also travels out to more rural areas to meet with interested groups there.

Interviewer: Can you just explain what the [ideal] programme is?

Programme coordinator: [Ideal programme] … I actually pulled out my brochure [Laughter] 'cause I thought how am I going to describe this? So I'll give this to you. It's about first contact, it's about connecting people who are living with the disease either personally or with a family member, making that first contact with the [advocacy organization], becoming connected so that they are able to learn about resources, services, information about the disease and then are able to make informed choices. The two pillars that I personally feel are really important about the [ideal] programme are the direct referral, so the referral comes from the healthcare professional or community person, the onus is not on the person that is dealing with the disease. The onus is on the professional to identify that this family could use some help and they make the referral and then I contact them. So that's the one thing that I think is really critically important. The other thing that I think is really important is the follow-up. There's an 18-month follow-up. So I make the initial contact, have contact again in 6 months, 12 months and 18 months, which I think is really important in dementia care because things change so much over time and ultimately people would be referred early on in the diagnosis. (Interview transcript, programme coordinator)

In this first account we hear from a key informant responsible for connecting with people recently diagnosed with dementia. She works in between primary care providers and a disease advocacy organization. The priority for early diagnosis is offered within the justification of the programme, and there is no sense in this account that there is any controversy regarding the value of early diagnosis. Also of interest here is the implication that in relying on a referral from the healthcare provider, association with the ideal programme is not something the person with dementia is required to buy into. Rather, the programme is brought directly to their doorstep by this programme coordinator.

Despite all these apparently ideal features of the programme, the programme coordinator turns the conversation onto a less clear pathway that opens up alternate ways into her programme – and one that perhaps occurs more often than not:

> 'People don't tend to be diagnosed, I find, until middle stage. So it's not so early in the diagnosis. … There's often some sort of a crisis, I find. I find diagnosis actually occurs quite late, which is so unfortunate. There's often some sort of a crisis where somebody forgets something, something fairly significant happens like there's a car accident or somebody gets lost and is not able to find their way home. There's always something quite significant, I find, or you know, burners get left on or just increased agitation, sometimes aggressiveness. I find there's usually something quite serious that occurs and that's when people start to investigate.'
> (Interview transcript, programme coordinator)

The significance of the sort of events enumerated by this key informant are stark: car accidents, seniors with cognitive impairment being lost for minutes or hours, stove tops left on with personal injury or fire a possible outcome. If these are the events that more often bring people living with dementia and their caregivers into contact with support services, they are very different than those anticipated by the ideal programme outlined earlier. Rather than a primary care provider, a person may more than likely be initially identified as needing help by a police officer, a neighbour or a first responder. When these are the sorts of events that bring a person with cognitive decline to the programme coordinator's attention, a diagnosis now occurs at a much later stage and, she tells us, this "is so unfortunate". The benefits of the work of those who have developed the ideal programme are, in the her view, much less useful now to the person diagnosed with dementia at this later stage in the development of the disease.

This account offers a view of two ends of a spectrum in the everyday experience of dementia in the community: first, a programme designed to offer stability for families facing the early days following a diagnosis of a long, progressive disease; and second, an image of chaos that this informant suggests is perhaps the more common circumstance for both the allocation of a diagnosis as well as the opportunity for her to draw people into the ideal programme. Of note in both of these scenarios, however, is the importance of what we call practices of identification. Whether through the more stable route of referral from a primary care provider who has made a diagnosis in the office early in the trajectory of the disease or through the perhaps more common route of a person becoming injured following a car accident, for instance, the efforts of managing the problem of dementia rely on being able to identify people with the disease – to separate them out from others and to get them placed on a trajectory that is said to be full of "resources, services, information about the disease (so that they are) … able to make informed choices" (interview transcript, programme coordinator). All of this requires an informed 'reading' of individual and family situations to be able to make sense of the signs of dementia – as such, this programme coordinator exemplifies the semiotic effort of instituting forms of social stability (for example, a diagnosis of dementia; hooked into the ideal programme) linked to material distinctions.

These sorts of social stabilities are made manifest at the local level through the sorts of activities described to us by this programme coordinator. In our interviews with other key informants, we found how such stabilities operate in relation to wider strategies designed in other locales, and we now move on to those.

Convening for coordinated action on 'navigation'

Our next narrative is provided by an executive director who works for a leading dementia advocacy organization. She describes one of her organization's key goals: being a regional convenor to "tackle some of the really difficult issues around dementia" (interview transcript, executive director). She signals that there are several "players" in the region. The agency she represents is a leader among those agencies. The executive director describes some longstanding issues associated with dementia that she and the other "players" have been dealing with:

'I think, you know, if I go back a few years, there's many of us who work within this area that felt there was a lack of coordination. You know, there's a number of players who were contributing to dementia in the community but we were often working independently. We weren't sure what each was doing, so we saw a need to bring people together so we could get a better sense of what we're all doing, you know, improve communication and improve coordination and that's what initially brought us together.' (Interview transcript, executive director)

This key informant positions the challenges she faces in historical terms. She casts her mind "back a few years" to identify the key problem: "lack of coordination". Rather than focusing directly on issues confronting people living with dementia and those who care for them at home, this key informant locates the need for greater coordination as an interest of the collective: "we saw a need to bring people together so we could get a better sense of what we're all doing, you know, improve communication and improve coordination and that's what initially brought us together." This is not the end of their work, however.

What we learn as the interview proceeds is that this key informant engages representatives of the independent agencies in a strategic planning process where priorities for dementia care in the region are identified. Using a mapping methodology, the group develops a set of priorities and associated action items. The key informant tells us "… navigating the system is a tremendously challenging issue" (interview transcript, executive director). When asked what it is about "the system" that makes it so challenging to navigate, she struggles to offer a response. Here we point back to our analytic approach where we distinguish between what Giddens (1984) refers to as accounts arising from discursive consciousness and those arising from practical consciousness. Bringing independent agencies together to produce coordination so as to reduce the challenges of navigating a complex system reflects, we argue, an account from discursive consciousness. This series of linguistic moves is not difficult for her to offer us as an account of her work.

However, when we press further to learn more about system navigation, she experiences more difficulty. Our question seems to be placing her in a position where she has to dig deeper into her practical consciousness for an account. Further detail from the transcript illustrates the consequences of the executive director's reflexive monitoring of our questions. Please note that, throughout the book, ellipses in parentheses (…) are used to distinguish between ordinary ellipses – which are pauses in speech – while those in parentheses indicate text removal. We do this both to reduce the length of the transcript segment, as well as to add clarity to the account.

Interviewer: And what does navigating the system mean?

Executive director: When you're first diagnosed, where do I turn, what resources are there for me? It's a very complex … the health system is very complex. How do I access some of the resources available through the health system? Where do I even begin? So I think that, for families, it's very challenging. In-home supports for families to keep them healthy and strong can be very challenging. Access to respite for family members can be a challenge for people too … social isolation is a significant challenge.(…)

Interviewer:	What do you think it is about this situation that creates problems? What is it about that situation that makes it such a challenge for families?
Executive director:	I think there's a stigma associated with the disease and I'm not sure if you've seen the Alzheimer's Disease International Report from 2012? It's about stigma. It really, I think, paints a very clear picture of what the stigma is about. So often there's denial. So families may isolate themselves because they don't want their friends to know. There's a bit of embarrassment and denial or alternatively, friends don't know how to communicate now either, relationships have changed. So those changing relationships, I think make it very challenging for people. It makes it challenging for the family members too because over time it may happen that the person you're caring for doesn't know who you are, so your relationship has changed and that can become very difficult.(...) Once you've moved past you're requiring more support, so you're requiring home care, other living arrangements. It's just, they don't know where to start, right? And when to start. So what are those key identifiers for them that mean it's time to transition? (Interview transcript, executive director)

In this lengthy segment the executive director moves through a series of ideas to try to offer us an account of navigation that she hopes will do the work of carrying her meaning. She suggests that families have a lack of awareness of the help that is available. Referring back to the account offered by the programme coordinator earlier, this is a similar justification for her bringing the ideal programme out to people rather than relying on them seeking out information themselves. The executive director also points to the idea of stigma as being a problem faced by people diagnosed with dementia. At the core is a notion of families being lost, not knowing 'where to start' and 'when to start' the transition from everyday life to a time when help and support from the community is needed in order to care for a family member whose cognitive ability is changing. This is what is required for navigation to be accomplished: families need help to know where to start and when to start to seek help for their cognitively impaired family member.

Once dementia has been stabilized through a diagnostic process and stable programmes can be performed, including visits equipped with a compilation of informational resources, a strategy such as 'navigation' emerges, representing a 'material inflation' (Law and Mol, 1995, p 275) that links with other materials to create social shifts.

Extending navigation beyond human actors

If we take up the dementia-as-catastrophe narrative in a serious way, relying on individuals to carry information out to people diagnosed with dementia will soon falter as being too costly to sustain. In our next narrative, we hear from a programme director – someone responsible for implementing programmes for the advocacy organization. The programmes implemented within this team fall under one of two categories: education for family 'care partners', and organizing support groups and in some cases individualized support provided through phone and email contact. These efforts are accomplished through the introduction of an electronic portal. The programme director explains how the portal works:

'Our focus is that individual and the family, which is why with our [online portal], we have the three portals and we were very specific in designing that. So one of the portals is for people who are in the early stages of dementia. So the screens look very … not really different but they're much more simplified, they're less cluttered, maybe that's the term I would use, than, say, some of the web pages that you would use as a family care partner. So, and then the other one is just a browsing one for people who are interested, but on that we have all of our family learning pieces. So it's called [name of learning programme], which goes from pre-diagnosis to death and so we utilize various expertise, you know, we have an OT [occupational therapist], we have a geriatrician, all different kinds of experts that would come and speak at each one of those in, I guess, in-person sessions where in rural [province] that's not often possible.' (Interview transcript, programme director)

The portal functions in response to what we described in Chapter 1 as an overdetermined image of dementia. Anticipating significant need for information and access to services, it organizes those resources in a way that would be available to anyone logging in. It also serves to extend the efforts of people such as the programme coordinator whose account appeared earlier. The portal performs practices of identification: first, it sorts people into categories (for instance, those with early-stage dementia, family members and members of the general public seeking basic information about dementia); and second, it provides specific kinds of information under each of those categories.

While the portal can extend the effects previously delegated to workers associated with the ideal programme and support the strategy of navigation, problems with navigation are also experienced by this programme director:

'Last week in a meeting I was at, we were talking about system navigation and somebody made the comment that really system navigation is a unicorn. It really doesn't exist and no one really knows what it looks like.(…) Part of the challenge is, I find that even people within [health authority], they don't really know how all the system works either. You have your areas of speciality and so I guess like for us, as the [advocacy organization], I've often suggested we're a bit like the listing on the main floor of an office building, you know? If this is kind of, you've identified this, we can kind of be that listing of how do you get to that … whatever office it is.' (Interview transcript, programme director)

Here is an instance of a stable strategy, navigation, suddenly appearing a little more shaky. Some people with whom the programme director interacts argue that "navigation is a unicorn. It really doesn't exist". The programme director seeks to resolve the controversy in her account to the interviewer by reiterating how widespread the problem of understanding the system is: "even people within [health authority], they don't really know how all the system works either." In telling us this, it seems she is propping navigation up as a matter of recursive and reflexive material distinction (Law and Mol, 1995, p 275). She circles back to point at those working in the very system that needs to be navigated to show how, "people within [health authority]" may not see navigation as an issue. In doing so, and while trying to reinstantiate navigation as a core priority that everyone should share, she separates herself, as a representative of the advocacy organization, from her colleagues in the health authority. She reasserts the advocacy organization's central role in supporting navigation, citing its similarity to a board on the main floor of a building advising which offices can be found on each floor.

Within these last two accounts, we can point to the way in which an advocacy organization positions itself in relation to community-based support agencies as what Moreira (2017, p 5) refers to as 'knowledge making practices'. By developing associations with 'independent' agencies with an offer of enhancing coordination, the advocacy organization makes itself larger and more powerful than what it might be on its own (Latour, 1984). It is enacting power through its associations of people who attend meetings and contribute to the development of materials like the portal, designed to organize the wider population who are doing the work of dementia care at home in communities. The controversy over the 'reality' of navigation signals a limit to the ability of the advocacy organization to claim primacy over dementia as a field of influence. While the advocacy organization and the independent community support agencies have gathered together as a knowledge-making institution to organize dementia care, their strategy of social change aiming at early diagnosis, attachment to the ideal programme and a promise of navigation across the length of this progressive disease shows some sign, in these 'here-and-now' encounters (Law and Mol, 1995, p 275), of being a bit unstable.

Patchwork 1: "We'll make it work, don't worry about it"

The performative effects of material distinctions, developed through practices of identification and then elevated as strategy into social change, as told by our key informants thus far, show how populations are divided up, and resources are gathered together and made accessible through the ideal programme or the electronic portal. Navigation is offered, either through people associated with these programmes or through the electronic portal itself, so that those living with cognitive impairment are assisted in navigating towards the support they will need to continue to live safely in the community. But it is not just colleagues from the health authority that throw the rationality of the ideal programme and navigation into question. The programme coordinator who offered the first account told us about an incident she had recently dealt with that did not seem too much out of the ordinary:

> 'A gentleman just drove up here the other day and he came in to see me and he was telling me that his wife had dementia and I realized that his wife was still sitting in the car. So I just said, "I think you need to ask her in. Like, bring her in and we'll just … we'll make it work, don't worry about it", because he had left her in the car, and that kind of thing makes me very nervous, somebody unattended, you know, especially if they're further along in the dementia.' (Interview transcript, programme coordinator)

Despite the fact that the programme coordinator works as part of the ideal programme, accepting referrals from primary care providers, linking people up to the advocacy organization and following them up at six-month intervals following referral, she is *also* present and available to provide much more immediate, direct support alongside her formal work role. The scenario she shares with us here could be read as an instance of failed coordination – the very purpose of the ideal programme. But has it failed? Noticing a potentially dangerous situation, the key informant's account suggests that she takes action by instructing the caregiver to bring his wife into the office where she will assist them to "make it work". This seems to us to be an instance of patchwork.

Law and Mol (1995, p 275) argue that patchwork relies on a 'sensitivity to the possibility that social and material relations don't add up, semiotically or strategically'. Acting very much in the 'here and now', the programme coordinator looks past the man at the door to a woman she decides is very likely his wife, the very person who is the source of the trouble for which he is turning to the programme coordinator for help with. The programme coordinator makes a quick reading of the situation: here is someone who knows he has trouble but who does not understand the scale of the trouble, so much so he leaves his very vulnerable wife in a car on her own. Anything could happen. She could release the brake and roll away in the car; she could leave the car and wander off – all the sorts of things that an early diagnosis would aim to reduce the likelihood of. And so the signs are not adding up to a situation that would suggest this man and his wife are part of the ideal programme and know how to navigate the system. They did not seek help earlier – they are seeking help now. She invites them in and reassures him that she will 'make it work' for them.

Patchwork 2: 'What else are you going to do?'

Most of the accounts we heard from our key informants told us about the dementia problem as primarily located in the person living with cognitive impairment as the focus of action and practices. It was that person who needed to be seen by a physician or someone who could diagnose dementia – early, preferably – so that they could become associated through strategies of navigation with information and services such as those offered by the ideal programme. But one of our informants told us a different story. In her story, it was the caregiver who was the focus for her work. This informant's role was as a caregiver support therapist. She told us about how her role had come about:

'I am a caregiver support therapist with [health authority], a new position that was created about, well almost three years ago and I'm participating in, actually, a new programme with home care. They wanted a dementia care team, which consisted of a case manager, who's a nurse, occupational therapist, a caregiver support therapist, with the opportunity to bring in other specialties as required into that team. The idea was to support the whole family in the context of dementia, recognizing that just interacting with the client, we weren't always getting the right information and as the disease developed, there were problems arising in knowing what was correct and incorrect and in response to the caregiver and if the caregiver wasn't doing well, then the client was not going to do very well.' (Interview transcript, caregiver support therapist)

The caregiver support therapist opens up a new possibility here: in her role as someone trying to offer support to the 'whole family', sometimes it is necessary to separate off the person living with dementia from those family members providing care. Someone on the team had recognized that, in maintaining a focus on the person living with dementia, as directed by another central strategy, that of "patient-centred care", the team was not "always getting the right information". And so, the concept of the 'whole family' becomes elevated, thus creating the opportunity for the caregiver support therapist to focus on those people caring for the person living with dementia at home in the community.

Asked whether it was fair to rely so heavily on family caregivers in order to achieve the aims of community-based care for seniors living with cognitive impairment, the caregiver support therapist responds:

'I think they need to be at home, predominantly, but I think we need more care, I think we need more supports around it. I mean, (a) we couldn't do it in institutions and that would be impossible, but how do we create more support around it as this thing gets bigger and bigger? So, and some families maybe not. I don't know if I would say "fair", it wouldn't be a word I would use. What else are you going to do? I mean these people are getting sick and in some cases, families do amazingly well, but we need somebody behind them saying, "How are you doing?" and "Is it going okay?" you know? "What is the dilemma for the day? Is there anything that we can be providing?"' (Interview transcript, caregiver support therapist)

Offering her account from the position informed by the overdetermination of dementia, of the 'looming catastrophe' of a major public health issue, the caregiver support therapist response initially endorses the organizational goal of keeping people diagnosed with dementia at home: "we couldn't do it in institutions ... that would be impossible". But at the same time, her comments attest to a recognition that there is a need for "more care ... more supports around" the policy of delaying institutionalization.

We are inclined to name the approach described here by the caregiver support therapist as an example of what Annemarie Mol (2002) calls 'inclusive'. Rejecting the institutionalization of people living with dementia does not have to mean that the person and family living with dementia are unsupported by professional care personnel. But perhaps pointing towards what we noted at the outset as a marked 'underdefinition' of the full scale of the dementia problem, her inclusive question, "What else are you going to do?", might signal that just what families might experience as supportive is not necessarily evident, even when a caregiver support therapist can focus on the caregiver who can offer the "right information".

We think it is interesting that the caregiver support therapist does not become overwhelmed by the overdetermined problem of dementia. And notably, she does not fall back on the need to better define the scope of the problem. Instead, she recognizes that some families do not require that much help. And, as she finally responds to the key question that was asked – "is it fair to ask this of families?" – she turns the question over – fairness may not be the most appropriate context for thinking about this problem. Instead, she asks the more inclusive question: "What else are you going to do?" And follows this up with questions about the hyper-local issues for the caregiver: "What is the dilemma for the day? Is there anything that we can be providing?"

Discussion: identification, strategy, inclusion

In this chapter we have focused on the work of professionals as they think about and implement programmes designed to stabilize a particular notion of dementia that aims at identifying people living with dementia early, and then offers them information and support to help them remain living at home in their communities. We have drawn on the interviews with key informants to illustrate practices of identification used by these professional caregivers. The practices, we have argued, rely on a semiotic heavily influenced by a 'looming catastrophe' framing of dementia. The key informants we spoke with rely on their performances of distinctions between people who are cognitively well and those who have cognitive impairment, members of the medical community, people who work in other areas of the health system and those who work in the community, in order to design strategies that recursively frame the dementia care system in ways that can be treated as stable. Programmes designed to find cases of dementia early and navigate people into programmes offering information and services form the majority of the work they described for us.

A particular form of dementia is brought into relational effect through the implementation of what was described as an ideal programme. People become diagnosed early, families are informed of resources and are followed while living in the community; someone, somewhere, determined that a six-monthly check-in would suffice as support, so support is also brought into relational effect here. Navigation, dementia and support are all operating together to create social stability and changing unruly demands associated with the 'looming catastrophe' into something much more orderly; and the orderliness of the strategy recursively and reflexively creates demands associated with dementia – navigation and support – further strengthening the delivery of navigation and support to address the dementia problems identified by people working in the programme.

But, as we have shown, that strategy is quite unstable: navigation may be a "unicorn", people don't get diagnosed until later, and anyway, it turns out that it is the caregiver who needs help. The person living with dementia cannot really offer the right information. The caregiver support therapist told us that people living with dementia need more support around them; you can go in planning on implementing the ideal programme, but in the end, you just deal with the problem that's there today, which suggests the ideal programme likely does not actually address these issues.

Here we begin to see the complicated terrain that people living with cognitive decline and the families who hope to support them encounter in the health and social support service sector. The requirement voiced by journalists and other community care advocates to manage the 'looming crisis' is very loud. Often the first thing that is done when such loud demands are made is to make a plan. But these are plans designed at a distance, far away from the singular worlds and myriad troubles that people living with dementia and their families occupy. When you start to listen to those troubles and add them up, you can become overwhelmed by what people are contending with and the strained possibilities of doing anything that would be helpful to more than one person. And yet, dementia *demands* the attention of those with responsibility for financing and planning institutionalized health services as well as community-based responses to support those ageing in the community. Those in positions of authority must *do* – and be *seen* to be doing – something to address this problem. Despite the fact that they are dealing with a condition that may evade planning (Gronemeyer, 2017, p 20), and for which specific solutions – especially those that frontline workers have independent authority to implement – are hard to come by, the key informants we spoke with talked about developing strategic plans, information portals, staffing projections and innovative programmes – all designed, so it would seem, to respond to the 'looming catastrophe'. Remarkably, our key informants did not seem overwhelmed by the 'rising tide' of needs (Dudgeon, 2010).

What makes this set of circumstances interesting to us is that the key informants we spoke to could offer us an insight into both the nature of the problem associated with population ageing and the demands of seniors living with dementia – but also, and importantly, how they go about responding to those problems. Nowhere did we come across a key informant who did not take seriously the fact that dementia is a real problem for those living with it, whether as the person diagnosed or the family members tasked with providing care for that person. But also, we did not encounter key informants who were immobilized by this 'looming crisis'. Despite the lack of definition and clarity about this problem, they seemed to have well-practised strategies they could deploy in the particular case. So, even though what often appears to us as stable (that is, national dementia plans, the ideal programme and so on) shows itself as unstable at the level at which it is proposed to have effects, these key informants evince an understanding that it is possible, that despite the tremendous work and power of plans and programmes, these may not really 'hang together as a whole' but rather are necessarily patched together in multiple ways (Law and Mol, 1995, p 286). This brings us back to our earlier question: is patchwork evidence of system failure? Or is it, perhaps, something of an inclusive failsafe when conditions permit its operation? From our interviews it seems, at least at times, to be the latter possibility and, we would argue, this may be a better option. When conditions permit, 'partial and varied connections' may be made between people, programmes and plans, and support for people living with dementia and their families can be woven together 'like bits of cloth' and turned into a 'whole variety of patchworks' (Law and Mol, 1995, p 290), attentive to that helpful idea discussed earlier, "What else are you going to do?"

3

How to support care at home? Using film to surface the situated priorities of differently positioned 'stakeholders'

We started our book with a description of 'traditional' narratives for understanding the problem of dementia for our communities. We have already noted that these 'traditional' or common ways of thinking about policies designed to address the problem of dementia frequently frame solutions in economic terms. With growing numbers of people affected by the disease, and with limited institutional resources for meeting that demand, the home is figured within policy documents as a location best suited – that is, most economical from a policy perspective – for people living with dementia. Our first two chapters have created opportunities for us to raise questions about this common formulation.

In Chapter 1 we pointed out how traditional economic formulations framing the problem of dementia might actually be excluding other, less traditional, less common, but possibly more inclusive, ways of understanding the problem of dementia. The near-exclusive framing of dementia as an economic problem means that very little space is left to describe the thickness of problems (Savaransky, 2018, p 217) associated with living, everyday, with a diagnosis of dementia. In Chapter 4 we begin to explore this thickness of problems by introducing readers to the families who shared time with us to help us know better what everyday life living with a diagnosis of dementia is like.

But it is not only in everyday lives in homes where thickness can be described. In Chapter 2 we presented a 'thick' reading of practices associated with policies that constitute the home as the 'best place' for people living with dementia to receive care. We showed how, with an interest in mapping the population for the purposes of gathering knowledge of the (economic) scale of the dementia problem, programmes designed for early diagnosis are created and mobilized in the community. But we also saw how unstable those programmes are. Despite common formulations of institutions as powerful, we saw how the ideal programme requires navigation through a complex system of health and social supports. And, as even personnel associated with those health and social support programmes recognize, navigation may be experienced more as a 'unicorn' rather than the everyday reality of seeking help. Instead of navigating that complex institutional landscape, some people are fortunate enough to meet a care provider who uses her or his discretion to "just deal with the problem that's there today".

Chapter 2 brings the work of planning to bring help closer to the people living with dementia in homes and communities into focus. Before we move on to describe what might be considered the other side of that equation – that is, the experience of receiving help from health and social services – in this chapter we introduce readers to a space for analysis that enables us to hear from a range of different actors, each of whom represents a unique perspective on our core interest: care for people diagnosed with dementia who live at home in their communities.

In order to draw out and show some of the 'messy differences' at work in the underneath of the problem of care at home, we made a film from our ethnographic data and then used this as a starting point for discussion in meetings with groups of people who could be said to have different stakes in the issues: people living with dementia and their families, direct service providers and policy-makers and researchers. These discussions represent the only time where we were able to bring all these parties to a table where they all saw, and responded to, the same set of practices (as presented in the film), and where we could engage in a discussion with them about their reactions, understanding and thoughts about what they saw.

In Chapters 1 and 2 we suggested that around the 'problem' of dementia in general, and care at home for those living with a dementia in particular, are gathered many different groups with differing interests and concerns. While this is unsurprising, an issue that remains undertheorized is the effects of these disparate interests and concerns among those involved in different ways in the problem of care at home. While we don't suggest that interests are singular or 'pure', and indeed overlapping concerns seem likely, it also true that there are longstanding challenges in reconciling institutional priorities of health and social care services required to be responsive to fiscal and political contexts, the exigencies of professional practices and the variable, changing arrangements necessary to everyday life at home. Such institutional priorities are evident in policy documents and programmes – such as the ideal programme described in Chapter 2. There are also, for example as noted in Chapter 1, well known and well documented frictions between family arrangements and those of formal care systems, which finds families at times reluctant to use services meant to be helpful or using these supports without experiencing them *as* helpful (Lyons and Zarit, 1999; Büscher et al, 2011; Keefe, 2011; Lloyd and Stirling, 2011; Stephan et al, 2018). Researchers studying systems set up to support families in different nations have identified a very similar range of concerns including, for example, that the relations between formal and informal carers are often unclear and subject to unexpected change (Dunér and Nordström, 2010), that formal systems' processes may impinge on usual family care practices (St-Amant et al, 2012), that receiving help sometimes requires complex negotiations on the part of family carers (Egdell et al, 2010; Egdell, 2013), or that programmes set up to help may actually have unintended negative consequences for family carers (Lilly et al, 2012). And within formal care systems themselves, researchers document struggles to accommodate conflicting values and imperatives such as rationing care while at the same time trying to respond to the diverse needs of families (see, for example, Lymbery, 2010; Da Roit, 2012; Glendinning, 2012; Rostgaard et al, 2012; Glendinning et al, 2015).

Although in this chapter we don't intend to deal with each of these problems, citing this previous research, and the ways in which it points to the effects of policy in the everyday lives of people living with dementia, helps to 'tell a story'. This is not a story of the economics of caring for people living with dementia but rather of difficult longstanding relations. This story suggests that much work has been undertaken to understand and improve care for people living with dementia and their families, and also that although there are tensions in the relations, many actors working on many fronts are trying to sort them out. And this is certainly one story that can be reasonably told because it is, in many respects, quite true. But, as Law and colleagues (2013) might say, it is not the only story even if it is a smooth one, telling of progressive effort to improve care through building knowledge of its more or less successful conduct. In this chapter, although on the one hand we contribute to the accumulation of this knowledge of difficult relations, we also try not to smooth things out too much, or to resolve the tensions that have been observed and analysed in previous research. Rather, our approach is to try to show that part of the story, or perhaps even another story, is the 'messy differences' that animate and constitute the 'underneath' of the issues at hand (Law et al, 2013, pp 173–5).

As noted earlier, as part of our research we made a film from our ethnographic data, a film that told and showed a 'typical' story of a family where one family member had a diagnosis of dementia. We shared this film with different groups with the intention of learning about how these different groups of participants made sense of the story from their different positions or relations to the problem of care at home. We just note here that some readers may have concerns that we identify this situation as a 'problem', but we suggest this without assuming that a problem is negative (Savransky, 2018). Rather, as Savaranky suggests, problems provoke thought, are 'that which sets our thinking, knowing and feeling in motion' (2018, p 215). Confronted with the difficulties a family found itself in, as shown in the film, each group's task was to determine both what was going on as well as to think about what could be done. This sense-making practice is important because of the ways that solutions proposed always depend on what the problem is thought to be. Or, as Savransky argues, 'problems are open, and they do not say how they should be developed' (2018, p 224). As in Chapter 2, we take people's contributions in these discussions as reflecting their practical and social knowledgeability (Schutz, 1946; Giddens, 1984; Fernandez, 1986). That is, people's experiences, ideas and commonsense expectations – rules and resources relevant to the task at hand – enabled them to develop and offer an account of what they were seeing.

Our use of a film to engage people in discussion can be thought of as an experiment or 'intervention', a scene of action designed to create conditions to render more visible, and hence articulable, the perspectives of groups representing key 'roles' in care at home for people living with dementia. We examine the accounts of formal care providers alongside accounts from family members and people diagnosed with dementia as they all considered a *common* experience of living daily life. Our aim was to investigate the ways responses of these different groups differed, and to consider whether such differences could tell us something about the nature of the problem each group understands themselves to be dealing with. In this way, our shared viewing of the film took the form of an 'experiment', used to 'provoke' responses that would enable articulation of the situated priorities of differently positioned 'stakeholders' in care.

About the film

The film, *Care Collectives: Reconsidering Care in the Community* (Ceci and Brunelle, 2018), was developed using the rich descriptive detail of our Field notes to tell a story. However, to protect the identities of our family participants we didn't want to make a film that simply told one family's story. Instead, we created a composite family, choosing characters and events from our Field notes that we thought reflected a more or less 'typical' family story. The scenes from the Field notes were chosen by the first author (Christine Ceci) and two research trainees, Holly Symonds-Brown and Harkeert Judge. As much as possible, we animated the scenes with dialogue lifted directly from our Field notes. We employed a professional filmmaker to direct the film, as well as four professional actors to play the main roles of John, Karen, their son and the doctor. All other roles were filled by volunteers.

The film tells a story of a fictitious couple – John, who has a diagnosis of dementia, and his wife Karen – across five 'scenes':

- Karen's attendance at a caregiver support meeting where participants try to 'problem-solve' their family member's troubling behaviours.
- Karen and John's outing to their grandson's hockey game, which shows some of the complicated preparations needed.
- Karen and John's visit to the geriatric assessment clinic accompanied by their adult son, where they are given advice about John's 'stage' of dementia and how to keep him safe at home.
- A home visit from a healthcare provider who, like the geriatrician, gives advice about home safety.
- And finally, Karen receiving a phone call from John's day programme informing her that he is being discharged from the day programme for behavioural issues.

Film is thought to be an effective medium to show, and sensitize people to, others' perspectives and experiences, with ethno-drama being an emerging strategy for knowledge dissemination (Ares, 2016; Rossiter et al, 2008; Speechley et al, 2015; Taylor et al, 2017). Here, we were less concerned with the knowledge dissemination potentials of ethno-drama, using the film instead to investigate if or how responses to the film among variously situated groups might differ, and how this might help us to understand better what is at stake in sustaining various relations to the problem of care at home. Understanding this becomes important if we consider, citing Savransky (2018) again, that problems only become actualized in the sense that is made of them, and part of this sense-making may be found in the production of solutions. That is, we get to know what the problem is by looking to the things that are done, or are thought should be done, in relation to it. In the world of policy-making it is very often those occupying positions of authority over the development of programmes who draw on their own knowledge of the problem without always having access to how problems are known by those living in these circumstances. Showing the film to different audiences created a critical opportunity for these differently positioned knowledges of the problem to be made explicit.

In adopting this stance we are influenced by Garfinkel (1967), who showed that everyday practices of accounting for social life are part of how 'social life' itself is accomplished (see also Marres et al, 2018, p 19). As Marres and her colleagues argue, 'if we want to really grasp social processes we must somehow *invite*, *persuade*, or ... *provoke* actors and situations to generate accounts, and to produce expressions and articulations of social reality' (2018, p 28; original emphasis). In essence, we presented the film as a way to generate such accounts with the events of the film posed as an open question – *this* is something that happens/has happened, so what sense might be made of it?

Ethnographic storytelling as intervention

The film can itself be understood as an account or expression of social reality; it represents one version of our empirical work, a storytelling event in the way that 'all ethnographic descriptions are story-telling events' (Winthereik and Verran, 2012, p 40). As a re-presentation of events that 'really happened', it follows a logic that works to show something about how it is for someone, somewhere, as a specific instance of the phenomenon of interest. The ethnographic story is thus generalizing or a generalization, in the sense that it 'counts' as an example of something in general, and in our case, adds to what we know about care at home for people living with dementia (Winthereik and Verran, 2012).

At the same time, while such re-presentations are generalizing in this way, they are also partial and located; they cannot, and do not, seek to tell a 'whole' story or present a complete picture (Winthereik and Verran, 2012). The ethnographic story shown in the film sustains a tension because it cannot be said to be either fixed or finished. In its relations with viewers, it is continuing to do something, asking, for instance, about what happens next or before or instead. Winthereik and Verran (2012, 49) theorize the ways that ethnographic stories are agential, re-presenting 'the world' in ways that are generative, or in ways that provoke new relations that can also be understood as interventions, 'many directions are possible and many things may follow'. As researchers and makers of this film we take a position, we tell a particular story, an instance of something perceivable as more general – but at the same time, viewers also take a position that shows up in the ways they work to see the story told as an instance of something, in saying what it means for them. Sustaining this duality is generative, and working with it enacts the film as an intervention. Viewers of the film, in saying what the film means for them and in filling in the gaps, are telling us something about the nature of the problem they understand themselves to be dealing with.

Processes for the 'film intervention'

The film intervention was comprised of a series of six discussion groups held with differently positioned 'stakeholders'. Participants were recruited by word of mouth through local networks of the first author (Christine Ceci) and her research trainee, Holly Symonds-Brown. The six groups were made up in the following ways: a group of six family caregivers, a group of eight people with dementia and their care partners who regularly met as a support group, three groups of community care practitioners and other service providers (25 people in all), and one group of six people made up of those engaged in policy, administration or research. The service provider groups included participants from disciplines such as nursing, social work and physiotherapy – and in all cases, their work involved direct contact with families. In all, 53 people viewed the film and provided their responses to our open-ended questions regarding what they made of the actions observed. As with the main ethnographic study and the interviews with key informants, informed written consent was obtained from all participants prior to beginning our intervention.

Each discussion group was organized around a primary role or identity creating relatively homogenous groups. In this way we took the groups to hold an at least *partially* shared angle of interest in the topic of concern, for example family members, service providers and policy-makers. While these groupings do make some assumptions about interests, it is also impossible not to 'group' in some way (Latour, 1991), and the groups did have an advantage of a shared, recognizable history in relation to actual care at home for people with dementia, as well as in research and practice. Our choices about groupings were also informed by other assumptions: that groups of 'peers' might respond more freely, that power differentials (that is, between families and providers) would be somewhat mitigated, and that such groups would indeed have some shared interests that would differ in important ways from those in other roles. At the same time, methodologically delineating groups is messier (Law et al, 2013) than our groupings make it appear, and we recognize that identities beyond the role via which the participants were invited to participate might also influence how the film was viewed.

The basic format for each discussion was to begin with a brief overview of the ethnographic project on which the film was based. We provided information about how the film was made. Discussion after viewing the film was facilitated by the first author (Ceci), and highlighted a few central questions: what do you see as making life easier or more difficult for the family in this film? How does the formal system connect with the family's arranging work? What does it do well and what does it miss? What changes might be made?

Each discussion lasted from between 60 and 90 minutes. To support an informal atmosphere the meetings were not audiotaped. Instead, while the first author (Ceci) facilitated discussion, the two doctoral students, Holly Symonds-Brown and Harkeert Judge, took detailed Field notes in an effort to capture discussion content, flow of conversation and contextual issues. These two accounts of the meeting were then merged to produce a single account, including, as much as possible, the actual words of the participants who were identified in the notes by numbers. In the interests of confidentiality, accounts presented here are linked only to the role of the participant (that is, family carer, case manager). The anonymized merged accounts were shared with participants (by email or mailed letter, depending on participant preference) seeking additions or corrections to the content of the meeting account. No changes were requested.

In analysing these finalized merged accounts, our main interest was to capture how, in light of their specific interests in practices of care at home for people living with dementia, participants made sense of our film. The analysis focused on what was said by the participants and from what position or identity (that is, family member, care provider). Taking an ethnomethodological approach, we read people's accounts as expressions and enactments of their interests and positionings (Wilkinson, 2016), and this tells us something about relevant features of their social worlds. In this way we may become oriented, as Schutz (1946, p 467) argues, to people's 'interests at hand'.

As well as offering a glimpse into the participants' lives, framing of issues and situated priorities, their accounts were understood as related to the groupings that located them as people in a particular role interacting with others in a similar role. That is, in asking them to respond as service providers, for example, the research processes also positioned them in ways that meant they related to one another during the discussion as members of their group. This may have produced some disciplining (cf Foucault, 1982b) effects in the accounts that we remained conscious of while making our analysis. We did not take this as problematic so much as perhaps underlining situated priorities for the group.

Surfacing situated priorities

As we saw in Chapter 2, there is a general understanding on the part of policy-makers and health planners that families and people living with dementia benefit from navigational assistance in their efforts to sustain a good life at home. Despite their efforts to create navigational aids, scepticism remains as to whether these are as effective as all the effort to create them would suggest. That "something must be done", however, formed part of each group's discussion. But in framing solutions to the situation illustrated in the film, the 'problem actualized' in conversations differed across groups, showing something of the practical interests at work in people's situated priorities. The use of the film to begin a discussion was helpful to see this process unfolding as, to begin with at least, we were all talking about the 'same' thing. In many respects, the movement of each group was towards making this indeterminate situation into a determinate one (Schutz, 1946), one understood or known, and about which something might be done. If we follow Schutz here, it is our 'interests at hand' that break up an undifferentiated field into zones of various relevances, with the zone of primary relevance being that part of the world within our reach that may be 'changed and rearranged by our actions' (1946, p 468). In Schutz's terms, it is our 'interests at hand that motivates all our thinking, projecting, acting, and therewith establishes the problems to be solved by our thought' (1946, p 467).

At the same time, while 'interests' at hand shape what is thought relevant, such interests tend to be multiple and intermingled, leaving us having to decide which of our disparate interests will be foregrounded in defining situations and looking to solve problems (Schutz, 1946, p 469). This latter point is important in considering different groups' responses to the film *as* different as the interests and concerns expressed by participants within the groups were varied. Many participants inhabited multiple positionings in time and in relation to the problem at hand, for example we had service providers who had also been or were currently family caregivers.

Recognizing that requirements to 'purify' condition all research, insofar as our methods have in some sense designed out some of the 'messy differences' we referred to earlier (Latour, 1991; Law et al, 2013, p 173), it is still possible, however tentatively, to impute certain patterns to our data and to see participants' responses as accounts instantiating those interests that had most relevance to the matter at hand, that is, their role in care at home for people living with dementia. The participants can be seen as making readings of the film that reflected their primary involvement in different roles or practices, organized by different understandings, sets of rules, goals, material resources and the relations made among all of these (Nicolini, 2012). It is these patterns that we drew from our discussion notes, and with the limitations noted earlier in re-presenting these, we suggest that doing so shows something of what, from various positionings, are the most important problems to be looked after.

Reading events in the film: the 'plight' of the caregiver

The film told a story in five scenes, compressing events that would have taken place over many months into 23 minutes. This created a certain intensity for viewers, particularly for people living with dementia and their families. Indeed, the first thing we heard from family participants was about the 'overwhelming-ness' of the everyday. Family participants expressed a great deal of empathy for the caregiver in the film, seeing her as very isolated despite all the usual support (that is, home care, a day programme, binders of information about resources) shown as being in place: "She is also in an overwhelming position, I mean, like all of us here have experienced. It all seems to go back to her" (family group).

What they seemed to see, and relate to, was an experience of being fully responsible as both 'caregiver' and 'coordinator' of care. In contrast to understanding offered by the service provider groups, family participants suggested that the caregiver had enough 'information' but that there were overlooked complexities in actually being able to use this resource. We read this as a difference in the experience of being given or having information and the actual work of using it, including the idea that it matters who you call: "Having information doesn't tell you who to call" (family group).

Family participants carried this view to their comments on the actions of the healthcare providers in the film, who, despite being seen as caring, were positioned as operating in a different sphere: "There is an assumption of healthcare providers that people understand the healthcare system and how it works ... this underlying assumption is there that people know where to go and what's available, as well as specifically what might help" (family group).

Drawing on her experience to relate to the caregiver in the film, this family participant described being told she was 'entitled to so many hours of respite care. But the thing is, you have to find out who to ask' (family group). We see signals here that refer back to a policy directive relating to navigation: knowing one could access hours of respite care but not knowing who to ask to give you those hours. Turning the notion of navigation around from a planning initiative designed and implemented by members of the healthcare system, these family carers present themselves as already experienced navigators of the health system, watchful for just these sorts of hints about available resources.

Participants who were family carers also seemed to have a different attunement to the kinds of support that might help a family like the one shown in the film, in the sense of noticing that their challenges were related to the practicalities of everyday life, and that there was not a lot of 'practical' assistance on offer: "You know, it's overwhelming, like everything you have to deal with ... there just seems to be not a lot of practicalities" (family group). This sentiment was also echoed in the other family group: "It was as though nothing of what they actually needed was given. It was like they were told they had to fit these parameters" (family group).

For example, in the film the family is cautioned that they must supervise John "24/7" – while all groups acknowledged this advice was common, for families it was particularly perverse: "I think you did a good job of showing the 24/7.... How is it even possible? I mean I was at the grocery store and getting him to take the cart back just behind the car ... he got lost" (family group).

Advice given to the family in the film was also viewed as somewhat misguided, for example being told John should use a commode at night: "Like, the commode thing was not helpful, it's not like he is going to remember to use it at night" (family group).

At the same time as the family groups suggested practical assistance was missing for the family in the film, they had few specific suggestions to the question of what would make life easier, except that: "There can't be set rules. People with dementia are different and the caregivers are different" (family group).

While the family groups were reluctant to offer 'solutions' for the family in the film, one family participant expressed ideas about broader system reorientation. The 'system', he suggested, is "housed in the medical model and maybe that doesn't work the best. In some cases, it may be better to understand what the needs of this individual and family are, and then fit the services to that" (family group).

There is a resonance here with the account provided by the programme coordinator in Chapter 2 who recalled inviting a carer into her office where she said she would help him "make it work".

In the suggestion from the family participant quoted previously, the timely responsiveness demonstrated by the programme coordinator of bringing the carer in to understand his needs, and fitting services to that understanding, reflects a desired approach in contrast to how help was reported to have been experienced.

Family viewers' positioning of the healthcare providers in the film as somehow missing the 'real' nature of what was actually going on for the family (that is, not enough support for the practicalities of everyday life) in some respects mirrors the responses of provider discussion groups to the caregiver's situation. These groups also expressed much concern for the caregiver in the film: "I see the burden of care, what it looks like for the care partner – everything is thrown back on the care partner" (provider group).

But here, the caregiver in the film was *also* positioned as not quite doing a 'good enough' job. In this case, it is the caregiver who is missing what is 'really' important: "I see a lot of caregiver burden. ... She is too stressed, so she isn't coping well. That's why when the day programme called and discharged him she panicked and called everyone. It's not like it was an acute situation" (provider group). Other members of provider groups expressed similar views concerning the caregiver's failure to 'be prepared': "Self-care was missing by the caregiver. She needs to be better prepared to deal with that situation" (provider group). Or from another provider: "Self-care could help in terms of how you plan and react to Plan B" (provider group).

From a positioning within "the system", provider participants showed an inclination to see that system, even while perhaps placing too many demands on the caregiver, as still doing its job. And even while they see that the caregiver is overwhelmed by demands, the solution offered is additional work for the caregiver: she needs to learn how to "self-care". Their tendency was to frame the problem in terms of individual coping. The focus on "self-care" in the discussion, and on rational preparation and planning for an "unknown" but apparently predictable future (and thus seeing "solutions" in terms of being prepared for the "trajectory of the disease", or helping clients to "map their journey" [provider group]), demonstrates something of the organized and organizing character of their own practices, even though it was also recognized that the experience of providing care is "not the same for the family as it is for us" (provider group).

Concern for the caregiver in the film was also present in the discussion with the policy/researcher group, again, with reference to an absence of self-care and the problem of isolation: "You get a lot of people not caring for themselves ... that self-care is missing" (policy/

researcher group), or "You can see a lot of social isolation for the caregivers of people with dementia. I hear a lot about how people don't know what to do with their loved one's dementia behaviours" (policy/researcher group).

Similarly to the provider groups, policy/researcher participants also focused on specific actors in the film such as the doctor and, also like the provider groups, framed the issues presented in the film in terms of *individual* attitude or behavioural problems of (ineffective) healthcare providers that might be corrected with better training and/or education: "The physician in the film ... she showed very little insight as to what is going on with the family" (policy/researcher group).

Their responses rarely framed the problems within the context of the wider system of care. Interestingly, the family groups were not specifically critical of the healthcare providers in the film, perhaps seeing them located in and constituted by that wider system of care.

'Trying to work it into life': marking time versus living 'in' time

In positioning or articulating the problem posed by the film there was a tension in all the groups between a medical picture of a dementia trajectory, something that proceeds in foreseeable stages, and everyday life with a disease that is uncertain, unpredictable and not necessarily able to be planned for. One participant living with dementia described the film as discouraging, relating this to: "The inevitability of that trajectory and what's going on and how long I'll last" (family group).

Or, as another viewer living with dementia said: "This may be hard to hear but finding out how long we have left and trying to work it into life can be hard. Figuring out what stages we are at – are we beginners, mid-termers, and what should we expect?" (family group).

Family viewers were well versed in the idea of stages – both relating to this and resisting it: "We also try not to dwell on the stages because they aren't the same for everyone, everyone is different" (family group).

There was a sense here that information about the stages of dementia, as discussed by the family in the film with their doctor, was a familiar part of medical engagement, but not necessarily helpful information in daily life with disease where differences among people and situations were posed as more important. It was only family participants who commented on the specificity of the arrangements of the family in the film ("I think she had a better arrangement with her son than most other families" [family group]), while at the same time noting that other families would have other arrangements.

The tension between a medicalized trajectory and everyday life with disease was also articulated in a discussion about how the family in the film was dealing or not dealing with 'reality', that is, with a problem (dementia) that needed preparation for what might happen next. These discussions occurred alongside comments reflecting the difficulty of doing this, a question, in a context of unpredictability and difference, of for what you would prepare. Observations from participants in the provider groups are illustrative of the way that the question often arose: "She's trying to maintain normalcy ... She's trying to keep life how it used to be" (provider group). Or as expressed by another provider: "I think they want a fix, because she's trying to maintain life despite the significance of those losses ... maybe that's why there's caregiver denial" (provider group).

When asked by the facilitator what the situation would look like if there was no caregiver denial, the participant responded: "Maybe she would have a Plan B for a more advanced scenario or more forward thinking to broaden her perspective instead of thinking of the now" (provider group).

Yet, at the same time, when pressed, this participant showed awareness of the difficulty of doing this:

'I guess people can't project their concerns into the future. Every day is a new day. Foresight is hard. Most people can't look at the future .... One day he can't put his jacket on, then he might be incontinent. Can you really be ready for that until you have to deal with it?' (provider group)

This latter observation is similar to those expressed in the family groups who also saw 'the wife' as "trying too much to keep things the same ... but you can't do that, you have to deal with reality, come to grips with our reality" (family group).

Where the two types of groups diverged, however, was in the strength of the provider group participants' assertions that planning and preparation were important and practically achievable strategies for care at home. This was linked to their own positioning in the care system as 'problem-solvers' for families: "We know the system and how it works ... for the family, they throw stuff at the wall and hope it sticks. They don't seem to think about the future. They pay attention to the right now 'cause that's where they are" (provider group).

Within the provider groups there was a tension between their focus on their roles as planners of care, in Schutz's (1946) terms, their zone of primary relevance, and the acknowledged difficulties families may have in looking too far into the future.

Two different and tensive senses of time appear here – time marked in (somewhat) predictable stages that can be planned around and prepared for, and time connected to incremental, sometimes surprising changes that are necessarily "worked into life" (family group). In thinking about the problems posed by the events in the film, a participant in the policy/researcher group seemed to capture 'time' in both senses: "Instead, why isn't it, why don't we say we will support you to keep going and then in times of crisis we can be there to support you … everyone's trajectory is so different … we don't actually know what's going to happen" (policy/researcher group).

Here, again, is the idea of the significance of the particularity of the person – while they have a diagnosis of "a" disease, for the person and their family it is not really "a" disease but rather something more like a series of changing challenges that may be difficult to anticipate or prepare for. Holding these different and tensive senses of time might well be the core challenge for policy-makers seeking to think otherwise about dementia.

Seeing problems of connection

As noted at the outset, in many respects the movement of each group in discussion was towards making an indeterminate situation into a determinate one, a problem about which something might be done. The provider groups ventured most quickly into problem-solving mode – seeing events in the film in a very similar way as described by the executive director in Chapter 2, that is, as highlighting a disconnection and lack of coordination in service provision. Solutions to these issues were difficult to articulate by these groups except in terms of what would be the opposite case, that is, better coordination, more information, more navigation: "I see a family unit but they aren't being treated as one …. Our system is so disjointed, it's not that it's not there but nothing really connects, there's a lack of coordination" (provider group).

The well-rehearsed discourse of healthcare 'silos' was employed in the provider groups to describe the problem: "Nobody is putting it together for them … it's disjointed … there's no linear connections" (provider group). Or as described by another provider: "The healthcare system is [made up of] such silos, day programme, geriatric clinic, home care – and no one talks to each other. As soon as you are out of there the door closes" (provider group).

At the same time, again echoing comments made by the executive director from Chapter 2 who convenes all the 'players' in an effort to improve navigation, the suggestion here is that: "There is good work done within silos – I don't think it's a lack of services, just a lack of coordination between them" (provider group).

Words used in the family groups, to describe what they saw in the film but also with references to their own experiences, echoed those of the provider groups: "the system" is fragmented, disjointed, procedural (family group).

Framing the problems of the family in the film in terms of lack of coordination of services seemed to lead (inevitably) to identifying a need for better system navigation in every group's discussion, underlining the centrality of this metaphor in dementia care. The idea of interconnectedness seemed crucial among all the different participants, with interruption in the flow of different kinds of communication a key concern. Here families and providers shared a similar framing of concerns in terms of planning and future-oriented thinking; however, any options expressed, such as standardized communication protocols, specified system navigator roles, navigator workshops for families or online web portals, seemed to be acknowledged by most participants as marked by the same contingencies currently making system "navigation" difficult. Providers themselves described being challenged to find and make the "right" referrals: "Services sometimes don't mesh well as things change for families. There doesn't seem to be a connection between them. ... The toughest part is the navigation" (provider group).

And for families, with knowing what would help, or even if the kind of help needed was actually (and practically) available: "Like in the middle of the night, if there is a situation there is no place to go to for help. ... Who are you going to call? Like ghost busters? No one is going to show up" (family group).

This latter point marks a divergence of family group responses from most of the provider groups' discussion, the idea that rather than a system that needs "tweaking", it is the "character" of available services that might be seen as a problem: system-driven practices (which the provider groups also recognized) are "system-focused ... there was no relational focus" (family group). The problem of connection seemed to play out in a relational way for families in the sense of missing a connection with an actual person who "knows" and "cares" about them, who will "show up". For providers, on the other hand, problems in connection were most often figured as a kind of system breakdown that pushes towards the specific kinds of problem-solving noted previously (that is, more navigation). But this, too, was in tension for some provider participants who recognized that they may actually be missing what is important for families: "We assume that they can handle the burden and focus on task things, so we lose the other things that improve quality of life. We miss the whole picture of what does this really look like for the family and the person with dementia" (provider group).

Supporting diverging interests

We see our film as offering commentary on everyday events in the life of a family where one family member has a diagnosis of dementia, showing an instance of what this everyday is made up of. The film sustains a tension because it is not fixed, it is open to multiple engagements and relations – in a sense, providing a lever that loosens and shows the kinds of commitments we may have (Winthereik and Verran, 2012). Our analysis of the discussion notes shows the ways in which various groups diverged in their accounts of the events the film presents, including different senses of what "practical" assistance looks like, how time and "trajectory" work, as well as different ways to explain the problems of connection. However, these are not divergences of which it could be said that one group's reading was more correct or closer to the truth of the film. Rather, viewers' responses to the film show something of what, from various positionings, appear to them as the most important problems to be looked after.

For most participants, the film initially seemed to be regarded as something that might give them information about how to approach this situation of care at home. For family viewers, however, the film didn't really give them much of this kind of information although there was appreciation for the "issues" it showed. Although they empathized and related to parts of the film, and in some respects had their own experiences validated, the film did not offer direction. When asked, they tried to think of ways events described in the film could be different, but their inability to frame "solutions" suggests a primary and/or lived awareness that each family's situation is really quite unique. Their reluctance to tell others how to "do caring" also stands in interesting contrast to the primary mode taken up by the provider groups who moved quickly to offering solutions. For viewers with a dementia diagnosis, watching the events unfold in the film seemed to be equally unhelpful – they both related to the film and saw themselves as different from its main character, John.

For the provider groups, also strongly empathetic, viewing the film led to much talk about how this family was not doing all the "right" things and how their situation could be improved; they were interested in but also critical of the family carer, perhaps reflecting an idea that there is a "best way" to do dementia care at home. In their roles, care providers are always required to have something to say about what to do or what may be done, and as a result have lots of persuasive language, more than families, to fill these gaps. For example, discourses of care burden, self-care, system navigation, healthcare "silos" and so on were readily recruited to explain the difficulties observed. The policy/researcher group seem to have an "overview", but were not 'in it' in the same way as the family or provider groups, although they did rely on the same discourses as the provider groups (that is, of care burden and the need to 'self-care') to explain the observed issues.

So, in their various ways, different things were most attended to by people in different roles. Family participants would not problem-solve for the family in the film, seeing difference, unpredictability and perhaps inevitability in the scenes portrayed. Provider participants, even while reflecting on the limits of their own practices, repeatedly emphasized that people's experience with care at home could be positively altered if only they were able to be more planful – which seemed to also be a way of implying that family care practices 'should' or could be more like their own professional care practices. The pervasiveness of this as an approach to helping support families is made evident later, in Chapter 6. In contrast to the benefits of this approach as suggested here by providers, families encountered significant difficulties as they consider taking on such roles.

Although families and formal care providers are related through their common interests in sustaining care at home, they do not necessarily have the same interests in common – a finding that is unsurprising given longstanding and persistent tensions in relations among formal and informal care practices discussed earlier in this chapter. However, it is not our position that such differences are a problem to be overcome or finally resolved. As noted previously, it is not surprising that different interests would arise from the different stakes people have in even a shared concern. At the same time, it may well be a problem to attempt to make these interests align. Here, we are thinking back to Bond's (1992, p 5) early analysis of the politics of caregiving and the 'inherent contradictions' he identified in desires to align family and formal care practices chiefly, it seems, through a strategy of 'professionalizing' family carers (for a more recent discussion, see Ceci et al, 2018a).

If efforts to align interests and practices are potentially problematic, how could family and formal care practices better relate? Philosopher of science Isabelle Stengers' (2019) recent work on an 'ecology' of practices helps to reconsider the question of how to think about interests that are both related and diverging. In Stengers' view, the analytic stance *not* to take in a situation characterized by diverging interests is to subject them to comparison, to make a case for one or another as good or bad, better or worse, true or false; in an ecological framing interests are expected to diverge. Comparing and/or aligning is not helpful because it implies (but does not always acknowledge) a set standard against which interests may be measured, as well as standardizing discourses that may impose 'irrelevant criteria' or categories that do not concern the people involved (Stengers, 2019, pp 184–5). Efforts to 'professionalize' family caring, or to import the kinds of strategic planning professionals are known for, may run up against just these kinds of issues.

Instead, again drawing on Stengers (2019), supporting families may be better served by allowing these family and formal care practices to diverge – that is, to sustain their own 'positive and distinct way of paying due attention; that is, of having things and situations matter' (2019, p 187). Strategic planning and having a sense of the 'big picture' matter for formal care providers; it would be difficult to do their work without this. Families may be less attuned in these ways, and their concern with the local and particular may be what is sustaining for them. These differences may constitute divergences that are integral rather than epiphenomenal, showing through practical attachments what matters for each practice or what the crucial concerns are. To insist on an alignment of interests between, for example, families and professional care providers, would eliminate one or the other as distinct practices, and this does not seem a reasonable way forward.

Rather than alignment, or, as Stengers (2019) says, 'harmony' between practices, she suggests another term from ecology that may be useful in this context, 'symbiosis'. Here, where there is relational heterogeneity, there are beings or practices that are related by common interests but that also diverge. But in symbiosis, events that have 'diverging interests … now need each other' (Stengers, 2019, p 188). In more human terms, Stengers describes this as a kind of diplomacy between practices where what is sought after is not alignment but various kinds of 'rapport', connections that are legitimately divergent but that communicate, if only partially (2019, p 189). Important to the concept of rapport, in addition to its partialness is that the 'creation of rapport is always a local, precarious event' (Stengers, 2019, p 190), with partial connections needing to be worked out again and again. From an ecological stance, questions raised in seeking rapport are not necessarily about the 'correct' thing to do but what might be *good* things to do, here, now. For those in diverse roles with an interest in care at home, including families, providers and policy-makers, it may be that rather than trying to find the 'best' solution or the best practice, creating a context that enables moments of rapport that allow for, or even foster, diverging interests is the more pragmatic move. It would be to keep at the forefront of providing and planning one provider participant's words: "it is not the same for the family as it is for us" (provider group). It is this last point that we delve more deeply into later, in Chapter 5.

In this chapter we described part of our study in which film was used as an intervention to provoke a discussion about the problem of care at home in the context of dementia among different groups of stakeholders. Our aim was to try to see, through these discussions, the situated priorities of different groups, specifically, how different positioning in relation to the issues of care at home shaped interpretations and discussions of the events portrayed in the film. Our analysis suggests that readings of the film were highly influenced by position, reflecting viewers' stake in the problem as well as their orientation to what might be done about it. The distinctions observed here add to our understanding of the longstanding and stubborn tensions that arise in relations among formal and informal care providers, which we argue are not so much a problem to be solved as a situation to be better worked with.

Acknowledgements

We acknowledge here the contributions of Holly Symonds-Brown and Harkeert Judge in organizing and helping to conduct the discussion groups, taking excellent notes of the conversations, and then helping to analyse these.

4

Negotiating everyday life
with dementia: four families

In the preceding chapters, we have taken steps along a pathway towards the central aim of our study. We have been laying some groundwork, offering context for the ways and places that the families and the arrangements they make for living with a family member who has been diagnosed with dementia intersect with other pathways followed by case managers, therapists and care workers in their daily work of offering specific care practices to others in the wider community.

We have always been most interested in the arrangements worked out by families in the context of caring for someone living with dementia. The preceding chapters have illustrated that these arrangements are not made solely by the families, but rather, they bear traces of influence from the formal care system at many points of intersection. We have focused on the work of those who have a formal role in supporting people living with dementia, not with a future goal of clearing the influence of those formal supports away from the practices of the families; instead, we take the position that these influences all become integrated into the everyday practices of the families.

And yet, as we have noted, while all actors in these stories may have a common interest in sustaining care at home, they may not hold the same interests in common. We believe that it is possible to tease these interests apart *to better understand* how they operate similarly and differently across unique family circumstances, and that the opportunities for expressing such understanding are enhanced by describing the practices of these various parties. Again, we want to underline that our purpose here is not to compare these different practices for the purposes of saying some are better than others when examined against a set of standards, but rather, to allow the family's and formal care practices to diverge.

This notion, drawn from Stengers' (2019) work examining comparison as a matter of concern, is not only a theoretical question we pursue in later chapters with a view to offering better ways for policy-makers and formal care providers to think about sustaining older people living with dementia. It is also useful in giving consideration to some important methodological issues when our research site is a family living at home, located in a community and networked with formal health services that both come into the home but also, at times, ask the family to come to the hospital, agency or office located elsewhere in the community.

When we think about the stories we have been told by families about their efforts to sustain themselves at home while caring for a family member living with dementia, and about what we have observed of their day-to-day practices, how can we think across these four unique families, noting similarities and differences among them, and the variable effects on their daily caring practices when intersected by formal service providers, but still allowing their practices to diverge? What are the research materials and analytic approaches that help us to engage in this work? How did we gather those materials and then transform them from the words, expressions and stories shared by family members into an interpretation that conveys the 'sense and significance that are wound up' (Jardine, 1992, p 55) in the families' words and stories?

Understanding: the 'play' of language

The analysis of our study materials arises from humanist traditions of interpretive research. Our work with the four families involved spending time with them early on to hear how they determined that their husband, wife, mother or father was changing in cognitive ability, the impact those changes had for the family, and then, as time progressed, we travelled with them to appointments – mostly with medical teams related to the diagnosis of dementia, but also on family outings. At each meeting we sat and talked with members of the family and recorded how they talked about what life was like each day – what was a struggle for them, what was working quite well, at that particular moment at least.

We paid attention to the language used by the families to talk about changes that, while noticeable, occur slowly over time, those changes occurring to family members they know well and deeply. They notice the changes but are not necessarily often called on to describe those changes. As we asked families to describe those changes, to talk about how life was before and how it is now, we were informed by the work of James Fernandez (1972) who writes about how ethnographers need to pay attention to the metaphors in use by those who have to explain what some*thing* or some*one* is like. Fernandez defines metaphor as 'a strategic predication upon an inchoate pronoun (an I, a you, a we, a they) which makes a movement and leads to performance' (1972, p 43).

In order to delve a bit deeper here, we offer an example from the previous chapter. There, one of the participants in a provider group who commented after viewing our film described their impressions of caring for someone living with dementia in a home setting in the following way: "I see the burden of care, what it looks like for the care partner – everything is thrown back on the care partner" (provider group). This short comment on the film evokes the weight on the family care provider – the burden of care carried by that person. And perhaps, more specifically, that care is 'thrown back' onto that person. By whom? What does that weight feel like? How heavy is it? Can it be borne? Who or what serves to relieve the person of that burden? What circumstances lead to further weight being 'thrown back' at you when you are already feeling heavily burdened?

When we read slowly and carefully, treating the words as we have here as 'strategic predications (that) make a movement' (Fernandez, 1972, p 43), we are in what Gadamer describes as the play of language:

> Whenever two persons speak with each other they speak the same language. They themselves, however, in no way know that in speaking it they are playing this language further … we adapt ourselves to each other in a preliminary way until the game of giving and taking – the real dialogue – begins. It cannot be denied that in an actual dialogue of this kind something of the character of accident, favor, and surprise – and in the end, of buoyancy, indeed, of elevation – that belongs to the nature of the game is present. And surely the elevation of the dialogue will not be experienced as a loss of self-possession, but rather as an *enrichment* of our self, but without us thereby becoming aware of ourselves.
> (Gadamer, 1976, pp 55–6, emphasis in original)

As we read the many hundreds of pages of the families' descriptions and explanations of their everyday lives, our dialogue with the text took us into this space of 'playing this language'.

Every day, as we go about our own lives, we all 'make sense' of what is happening around us and we adjust our course accordingly. We 'make readings' of the world. Interpretation, then, is not a new manoeuvre that we had to learn. But, because it is something we all do almost without thinking, as Gadamer says, 'without us thereby becoming aware of ourselves' (1976, p 56), in the course of engaging in an interpretive research project, we slow down in our work of making sense. And we pay particular attention to those stories that strike us as particularly meaningful. 'Interpretive inquiry thus begins by being "struck" by something, being "taken" with it' (Jardine, 1992, p 55). When something in a story strikes us in such a way, Jardine argues this is because those words are evoking in us something we find familiar, something we do 'not fully understand but somehow undeniably "knew"' (1992, p 55). Informed himself by Gadamer's work, Jardine notes that 'understanding begins ... when something addresses us' (Jardine, 1992, p 55).

Of importance here is the progression, the movement that such sense-making efforts generate. When struck by something vaguely familiar in a text, when that text addresses us, it arouses in us a new understanding of something already understood. And so, again returning to Gadamer, we follow an interpretive process of understanding where that process 'cannot be grasped as a simple activity of the consciousness that understands, but is itself a mode of the event of being' (Gadamer, 1976, p 50). It is the dynamic generating this new understanding that Gadamer is referring to when he speaks of the 'play' of conversation.

Gadamer's work is built from a somewhat radical notion that argues for understanding that does not require the possibility of actually knowing the other one is in conversation with. We can stand in isolation from one another and still engage in a language game intent on understanding. With his notion of the 'play' of conversation, Gadamer points to the work that two individuals enter into when in conversation, speaking back and forth, creating understandings in an intersubjective space fully understood by neither but shared by both. Understanding developed in such conversations is described by Gadamer as a 'happening' or, as noted earlier, as that 'event of being' (1976, p 50).

And this points to one further radical implication of Gadamer's (1976) work. If we follow his belief regarding intersubjectivity through, it brings us to his intriguing notion that:

> [A]ll understanding is self-understanding, but not in the sense of a preliminary self-possession or of one finally and definitively achieved. For the self-understanding only realizes itself in the understanding of a subject matter and does not have the character of a free self-realization. The self that we are does not possess itself; one could say that it 'happens'. (Gadamer, 1976, p 55)

The best we can do is to understand our own understandings better. At the same time, we do not arrive at a final understanding – as beings seeking understanding, we are always in play, always in motion towards another, further understanding in the next text we encounter or the next conversation we engage in.

This, then, is the place we locate ourselves as we enter into dialogue with these four families. In the next three chapters we offer our understanding of the stories of their lives of living with and caring for a member of their family diagnosed with dementia. Before moving on to those analytic chapters, we introduce the families to our readers. These introductions are intended to assist readers to engage with us in understanding the lives lived by these families.

Family 1: Colleen and James Miller

Colleen and James became involved with the research after receiving information about the study from a case manager at James' day programme. Our initial meeting was in February 2015. Our contacts included phone calls, visits and outings between March 2015 and the end of April 2015, when James was admitted to a long-term care setting. Contacts included going along with the couple to their grandson's hockey game, two visits with a geriatrician, two home visits and a home occupational therapy assessment. Phone calls and text messages were numerous as Colleen endeavoured to keep me up to date with a quickly changing home situation. A central concern for Colleen and the professional providers involved was the fear that James would become violent. This concern was the eventual reason for James' admission to a secure long-term care setting.

Overview

Colleen and James have been married for 44 years; Colleen is in her early 60s and James is 66. They have one son who is married with two children, and who lives nearby. James has four brothers who live in the same city, as do his parents who are in their 90s and still living independently. James and Colleen live in a large, comfortably furnished home in a quiet neighbourhood. Colleen says they have no financial concerns as she has been astute in managing their money. They had a fairly wide circle of friends, but many of these have dropped away as James' behaviour changed and he was no longer able to participate in their usual activities such as fishing and camping. Colleen suggests that those friendships were more about the activities than the relationships.

James retired from work two years ago; he managed a supply warehouse for the city. About three years ago Colleen says she started noticing changes in James – at first she thought he was 'being arrogant' or ignoring her because he wasn't responsive – then she thought it might be his hearing, but the hearing tests were normal. She noticed he was repetitive and that it was difficult to engage him in activities, and that when in a group, he didn't contribute to the conversation and didn't seem able to follow. She noticed these changes, as did her son and one of James' brothers. James himself seemed unaware of any changes. Colleen also mentioned that driving was becoming a concern in that he didn't seem to know how to get to familiar places.

Around this time, Colleen made a decision to change James' family doctor – in part, because the doctor had not noticed anything wrong with James, or did not seem to have a good grasp of James' medical history. For example, James had gone for his annual physical and had apparently been found 'fit', but he also didn't seem to know what the doctor had said to him. So Colleen went back with him to see the doctor. This is when she discovered that the doctor had little knowledge of James or the issues she was noticing. She asked her own doctor to take him on as a patient, and investigation of his signs and symptoms proceeded with a CT scan (which showed an old brain injury) and a neurological assessment scheduled for a several months later. At this point (and prior to a diagnosis), Colleen had completed the 'Empowering Caregivers' course at the Alzheimer's Society and was thinking James should be on Aricept® or Exelon® as she thought this would slow down the progress of his symptoms. She held off pushing for this until he had seen the neurologist as she wanted them to get a 'true picture of what he was all about' – but she did explain this situation to the receptionist at the neurologist's office and was able to move his appointment ahead several months. From this assessment, James was given a diagnosis of Alzheimer's disease. According to Colleen, James has no sense of the implications of his situation or any awareness of the ways she sees him as having changed.

Shortly after James was diagnosed, the family doctor felt James should no longer be allowed to drive – partly because while he could drive familiar routes, he could not find new destinations. There were also concerns that he could not safely process new information, and thus would not be able to respond appropriately to traffic cues. When told he couldn't drive anymore, he simply said that yes, he could, and described the places he could go – so they resorted to subterfuge, sending him a letter purportedly from the Minister of Transportation and hiding all the car keys. Next time he wanted to go out, he searched the house and found the hidden keys, which resulted in a confrontation between himself and Colleen – she had to call her son to come over to enforce the decision, as for some reason, James "listens" to their son more than to her.

This was the point, Colleen reports, that she realized that she was going to be fully responsible for James, and wondered if she wanted this and if she could handle it. She made contact with the local health authority and was assigned a case manager. One of the issues was James' age – at that point he was 62 and didn't fit in the right categories – but because they had a diagnosis and knew the disease would progress, they were set up with a case manager, and James was enrolled in a day programme.

At this stage, what was most important to Colleen was "information" – her assigned case manager was good at letting her know what was "out there" – at this time, they (she and James) did the 'Memory Plus' programme – a programme that is for both the family carer and person living with dementia – and Colleen was disappointed not to have more time during the programme for caregivers to meet separately as she was desperate for more information and felt the need to discuss caregiving tips with other caregivers. She says she wanted information – knowledge about the disease, what programmes were available for her and what resources – and was not interested in hearing about the experiences of other caregivers "managing their partners". She was also gathering and sharing information with her son and grandchildren. She says she needed information in order to be able to "deal with things". She says she wasn't dealing with things very successfully at the beginning, which she thinks was related to her occupation – she needed information in order to assess things, she needed that information in the right order, and she needed to know how things were going to progress, not knowing, then, that the disease takes all kinds of different turns. So they did those courses, James got into a day programme, she completed personal directives, goals of care, enduring power of attorney, updated her will, and dealt with Revenue Canada regarding tax implications given James' diagnosis. In some ways this kind of thing had always been her responsibility in the relationship – she describes with some disbelief a woman she had met in one of the support groups who was not able to make decisions about these things – but at the same time, she says the "ongoing-ness" of her responsibilities was tiring.

When asked what has been the most difficult for her over the past few years, she says it is simply getting James to do the things he has to do – for example, getting him to doctor's appointments requires her to hide the appointment in some more desired activity, like visiting his brother. James tends to simply refuse to do things, and getting around that can be difficult. But, as noted previously, their son is her back-up, someone who can convince James to comply. She also describes a "big struggle with medication" – but when she had it put in a blister pack, he began to take it with no questions. She doesn't know why, except maybe he can manage this himself – and now he will only take pills if they are in the blister pack.

At this point, James goes to the day programme three days per week, which is unusual, as patients are typically allowed a maximum of two days. Colleen got around the limit by arranging to have James attend two different day programmes, and the extra day is subject to space at the programme. She thinks that James needs three days a week because if he isn't at the programme, he sits watching TV all day; he seems happier if he can get out and about, at least a little. For her, she says the first couple of times he left, "I cheered out loud" – she uses this time to do errands, and says she's been told these "mini respites" are supposed to be about her – but when else is she supposed to get stuff done? When James is home, he's restless, and wants to be doing something. The activities the day programme provides – exercises and crafts – seem to be exactly what he needs. She says he's quite proud of his craft projects – but then says that she used to do crafts all the time, but James had no interest in those.

One of the troubles she has with James is that "he will listen to anybody else but me" – she thinks it is because they are together so much, and also because he has retained his basic social skills – he is polite to other people, but with her, he is rude, and sometimes angry. This turns out to be the biggest concern for Colleen. James is physically healthy, a tall, strong man – and sometimes she feels unsafe with him. So far, there have only been verbal outbursts – some of this has recently extended to other family members such as James' brother – which has validated her concerns. Up to now, she doesn't think other family members understood the extent of his anger and mood swings. This is why she is thinking about moving James out of the house to a supported living situation. Over the past few months he's become more restless, pacing, easily agitated, and harder to redirect. Her view is that this is only going to become worse, so she needs to be proactive.

One of the things Colleen learned through her caregiver support group is that sometimes people with Alzheimer's end up waiting for a placement through the hospital – she knows one person whose family member had been there (in hospital, waiting for placement) for seven months, and that after 30 days, the family has to pay the same amount as they would for a facility, but without the programmes. She is being proactive because she wants to make the choice, and not have someone else make the choice for them. So she's connected with transition services and has begun touring possible placement sites. First, though, the case manager assessed James, and then Colleen was given a list of appropriate placements to visit. In addition to this, she talks to many other people whose partners are in care in different locations. She says how valuable information from other caregivers is, citing the example of being offered a respite place at 'X' manor – which, she has heard from others, is a "hell hole". She refused the offer, preferring to wait for something available at another location.

James is pretty independent in many ways – he washes, shaves and dresses himself, although not always appropriately for the weather. They don't share a bedroom, but that had happened long before the diagnosis, as they have very different sleep patterns. When I ask if James wanders at night, Colleen says she doesn't really know as she takes sleeping pills. She started taking them because she was having trouble sleeping, attributing it to always needing to have one ear half open, listening constantly to what was going on: "I think it's like having a new baby where you've got that one ear open, constantly listening for what's going on". But she says she needs her rest in order to deal effectively with James. She also doesn't think she sleeps so heavily that if something were to happen in the night, she would sleep through it. She was advised by her caregiver therapist to have a lock put on her bedroom door, for safety, so she bought one, although she hasn't installed it yet. She could do it herself, but wants to get one of her husband's brothers over to help – while she is very independent and self-sufficient, and could probably install the lock herself, she wants to keep people involved and helping her.

The involvement of other people comes up in a discussion of what makes things easier for Colleen and James, and what creates difficulties – it is not straightforward. Just talking with James is challenging – she has had to learn not to ask questions that require him to make a decision, and how to ask him to do things but without "bossing" him. She says she's had to learn how to lie. She's had to learn how to schedule things in ways that match James' capacities – knowing he is more easily agitated in the afternoons. Even at the day programme, after lunchtime, the staff know they need to keep James away from certain other clients who "agitate" him. He tires, becomes agitated after two to three hours, and there is a need to get him back in his own surroundings, to prevent any outbursts. All of this means that other people don't know how to act around James, they don't know how to communicate with him, and Colleen says that as a result they (their friends) have pushed both of them away. People who were friends with 'Colleen and James' as a couple haven't been able to deal with the situation so she avoids them, doesn't talk about James' condition, doesn't answer questions. But she feels sad when she hears others at her caregiver support group talk about people's friends still being engaged. She describes a conversation with a friend in another city whose wife also has dementia and who is in long-term care – she asked him how often he visits, and further, when he visits is it for him or his wife? He told her he did it because people were watching him, and because they feel he hasn't done enough for his wife and shouldn't have placed her in long-term care. Colleen talks about this because she feels the same sort of pressure or judgement from James' brothers. They objected to her enrolling him in the day programme, and felt that "the family" could have come and checked on him a couple of times a day. For her, this tells her they have no idea of the nature of James' condition – they have 'opinions' about what she should or shouldn't do, but don't actually spend enough time with James to know what he's like now. One of the brothers did talk with the others to support Colleen, but that hasn't changed anything in terms of the actual help she receives from them. She says they don't seem to understand that James is different, that he can't participate in family gatherings in the same way, and that neither can she.

Colleen and James' involvement with the research was short but fairly intense as a "crisis" related to James' behaviour occurred early on which prompted what seemed to be an earlier than planned placement – although exploring placement options figured early in conversations with Colleen. Even in the first phone contact, initiated by Colleen, she spoke of a recent escalation in "aggressive behaviour" that had necessitated an increase in medication intended to "tamp down his temper but may make him more mixed up". What became clear from the first visit was Colleen's mantra – "ignorance is not bliss" – as well as taking multiple courses for caregivers and family members through the Alzheimer's Society, she had also completed a correspondence course through the University of Tasmania on "dealing with dementia". Through these activities, she had complied two 4-inch binders of information about resources available in the city, as well as information addressing legal and financial (tax) concerns. She also kept a notebook with a record of all her contacts with the formal health system (that is, case managers) – she says she maintains this collection of information because she is always asking herself "am I missing something?"

As noted previously, a "crisis" precipitated James' admission to long-term care. In a visit to a geriatric psychiatrist, Colleen and the doctor discuss placement as a "looming issue", with the key concern being James' behavioural issues, specifically that he can be "explosive".

During the visit Colleen brings out a notebook and begins recounting the number of incidents since the last appointment (about six weeks ago). She asks the doctor's advice as to what may be causing these issues, saying she is trying to problem-solve his "breaking point". This language is interesting because in a few weeks, an occupational therapist will visit the home, and part of her intention is to try to push James to breaking point to see how he responds (she does not succeed). The doctor suggests it could be a combination of things – fatigue, being out of his element, being challenged by an activity – these things may lead to "catastrophic reactions" – and that Colleen may need to shorten outings or have no outings, leaving James at home with supervision. The advice is to both accommodate James' changing needs and to continue to allow Colleen breaks from him.

The crisis leading to institutionalization occurs at James' day programme. His behaviour has become difficult for them to manage, and the day programme staff made the decision to discharge James from the programme. Colleen was very angry that this decision had been taken without consulting her – and because she had been unable to reach her case manager, family doctor or the geriatric psychiatrist for assistance. In her view, she says "a crisis hit and she expected people to respond" – she eventually called the case manager's manager, who indicated she would arrange a strategy meeting and try to implement home care companions for James so Colleen could still have some respite. She has reservations about companion care, worried that they would not be able to handle James. At this point, transition services contacted her and told her that he would be a priority placement. The placement offered for James is a secure unit, especially for people with dementia and behavioural concerns – Colleen says she is somewhat relieved that this placement has been suggested because if James had been placed in an supported living situation, there would always be the chance that his behaviour might result in him being asked to leave it. She accepted the placement offer and James is to move there in a few days; they will have the weekend at home to get organized. They will tell James he is going to camp. The weekend prior to James' admission was spent with family visiting, in a sense saying goodbye – Colleen says she felt like they were doing "last" things, for example, "this is the last family dinner we're going to have". Now that James is in care, Colleen says she wants to find a support group for people whose family member is in care – different challenges she says, a new philosophy, how to move on. In placement, James has "already hit somebody" – Colleen adds that now his family see that "it could have been me".

Family 2: Helen and Albert Baker

Helen and Albert are both storytellers – stories about immigrating to Canada as children, the changes and challenges of a new country including needing to go out to work at a very young age (neither stayed in school beyond the first six years of formal instruction). They have stories about getting married, working any sort of job, raising their large family, and building a business. Helen seems to contain suppressed energy, as though she is always excited. Albert, on the other hand is very sedate – he speaks deliberately and doesn't move about much once seated. There is a sense of stillness about him which may make Helen's "fluttery-ness" seem more pronounced.

Helen and Albert became involved in the research after hearing about the study at a caregiver support group Helen and her daughter Sandra had attended in August 2015. Our visits started in September 2015 and continued until April 2016 when Albert was admitted to a long-term care facility following a stroke. Our contacts consisted primarily of regular visits in their home, one appointment at the Seniors Clinic with a geriatrician, and after Albert's stroke, visits at the hospital. During the time they participated in the study, Helen and Albert continued to travel, taking two two-week road trips during the summer and autumn of 2015. Their travel ended when Albert's doctor recommended he give up his driver's license in December 2015.

Overview

Helen is 70 and Albert is 76. Both immigrated to Canada as children – Albert when he was 11, and Helen when she was 5 – from the same European country, although their families did not know each other. They both still speak their mother tongue, but with different dialects. Both seem to have grown up in fairly impoverished families, not attending school past sixth grade, needing to go out to work early. Helen, in particular, tells stories of how her family was employed as "beet pickers" when they arrived in Canada – their home was a "chicken coop" on the beet farm.

They have been married for almost 50 years and have eight children – five daughters and three sons, one of whom died young in an accident. Albert has had many jobs over the years, starting with farm work and factory work, and most recently owned and ran a religious bookstore, which one daughter now manages. Another daughter lives close by and is probably most regularly in contact with her parents. It is these two who seem to be the most aware of their parents' issues. Both daughters attended the doctor's appointment in November.

Helen and Albert's home is notable. It is an older home that started out fairly small, but by virtue of multiple additions over many years has become large and rambling. The most striking thing about the home is the "stuff" – Helen is a collector of many things including porcelain, dolls and other figurines – and everything is displayed somewhere in cases, on shelves. Entire rooms are devoted to displaying and storing these things. Helen says she began collecting after her son's death.

It is difficult to get a clear sense of events in talking with Helen and Albert. Most of the time we spent together, they tended to talk over each other and to disagree about details (in a friendly way). Part of the issue may have been that they disagreed about Albert's "dementia" – with Albert, especially when I first met them, not really seeing himself as having a problem, and Helen describing episodes or events that she tended to present as evidence of his having a dementia of some sort. The concerns seem to have begun about two years ago when Albert was still running the bookstore – one of his daughters worked in the store with him and noticed that he was misplacing orders and other papers. And then, about a year and a half ago, Albert had what Helen describes as a "stroke in his sleep" while they were visiting friends out of town. What he noticed the next morning was that his vision was affected – he was reading and could see clearly, but only part of a sentence. As a result of this event Albert apparently underwent a thorough medical work-up, seeing many different doctors, which he was somewhat perplexed by as he says he has been healthy his whole life. Apparently he is still "pretty healthy" as the only doctor requiring follow-up was the "geriatric doctor" – and no doctor has "come right out and said" he has dementia. But Helen insists there have been a lot of changes in Albert – she notices them but admits they are so subtle that somebody else might not see them.

The kinds of things she notices are forgetfulness, and that he can't be rushed or he gets confused (although she says this happens to her too). Albert agrees somewhat to "forgetfulness" – but describes it as "being rushed when I am already going fast enough". He sees himself as somewhat more forgetful – claiming that he has certain places for things, and if he puts things in the places he normally does (but not always), it is not a problem. He also notes that they have a big house with a lot of stuff in it.

During our first visit, I tried to get a sense of what the main concerns were, what had sent Helen to the Alzheimer's Society and caregiver support group. She says she went to the support group for information, that she knew "it" (dementia) was there, and what was she going to do about it? When she says this, Albert immediately objects. But Helen persists, saying that even though no one (that is, the doctors) has said it outright (which she finds frustrating), she knows. She had been hoping he might be able to take pills for his memory but he has refused. She also went to the Alzheimer's Society to see what is "out there" and what you can do and what they can do for you.

At this time, Albert was still working at the bookstore and so they had a family meeting, with all their children at the house, to convince Albert to stop working. They persuaded him to cut back on the grounds that his being there was causing problems for the daughter who ran the store (she was threatening to quit). Although Albert sees himself as having gone along with stopping work, he doesn't really think it was necessary. Near the end of our first conversation I ask Helen what she is most worried about – basically, she worries about what's going to happen from here on, "how is this all going to go?" – this is a worry because "it" went very fast over the past year, and she's noticed big changes. When I ask Albert what he is worried about he says it all depends "on what we have to attempt to do that is not normally done" – for example, going to different places or driving in the dark. Notably, none of these concerns have stopped them from planning a driving trip to visit family.

During one field visit with Albert and Helen, their daughter Sandra is present – she is a big part of their everyday life, frequently visiting, just dropping in or taking Helen out for coffee. There is a lot of talk about Albert's forgetfulness and the ways it is a problem. Albert resists this, saying that some people just get forgetful. Sandra comments about the ways he is doing things differently than he used to, for example, writing things down on little pieces of paper that then get lost. And Helen comments on how long it took him to sort through and pack a box of books. At the end of visit, Helen mentions that she and Albert are taking another trip and will be home in two weeks. This does not seem to be a concern for Sandra.

A month later Helen invites me for another visit, which proceeds similarly to previous visits – the three of us sit at the kitchen table and talk – we chat about their trip, they offer more of their family history, they share some of their values – for example, in talking about their work history, especially the hard life on the farm, they agree that young people today don't know what hard work is. They talk about how they organize their lives (Helen does the "inside" work, Albert the "outside" work – although they share a little more now). Helen spends a lot of time "keeping things clean" – which must be a lot of work, given her collections. She describes again her worry about Albert's forgetfulness – she is worried about the future because she knows things are going to get worse – and she will "have to do the thinking".

Prior to the next planned field visit, to go along with them to see the geriatrician at the Seniors Clinic, Helen sends an email saying that Albert has been in hospital – she thought he had a stroke, but it turns out it was a bladder infection that precipitated an episode of confusion – but he is home now, and the doctor's visit will go ahead as planned. Two daughters – Sandra and Alison – will also attend. The daughters are there, they say, because they are worried about both their parents ("mom gets muddled too"). When the doctor arrives, she identifies the purpose of their meeting to Albert as assessing the "performance of your mind" – from the family she seeks information about activities of daily living (ADLs), and frames things in terms of progressive decline. She brings up the issue of driving and enrolls the family in preventing Albert from driving.

The next time I see Albert and Helen is about five weeks later (after Christmas) – Helen has initiated contact and invited me for a visit "just to catch up". Later that week Helen sends me a note asking if the two of us could meet, without Albert. We arrange a date, but before that happens, I receive an email from Helen telling me that Albert has had a stroke and is in hospital. He remained in hospital from January 21 until March 10, and was then transferred to a long-term care facility. I visited them in hospital several times, usually having a short visit with Albert and then going to the cafeteria for a coffee with Helen. During the first visit Helen tells me that Albert had severe bleeding in his brain – she shows me a text message from her daughter that describes this as amyloid angiopathy. It took several days for the bleeding to stop. Helen is having trouble keeping track of everything going on and has handed responsibility for this to her children, who will keep her informed. The doctor has already suggested that going home will not be likely for Albert – he is not a "good candidate for rehabilitation" because of the dementia. His speech is currently affected and his left side is paralyzed. Helen is not hopeful he will recover much.

After Albert was settled in long-term care, I met with Helen and Sandra for a final conversation. Helen visits Albert every day, and one of her sons and two grandchildren have moved into the house. The purpose I set out for our conversation is what's been difficult, what's worked well, what it's been like for the family. Sandra distinguishes between the gradualness of her father's decline as being "easy to take" versus the drop (his stroke), which was really tough. One thing that was difficult was the healthcare system – this is a reference to his hospitalization.

Prior to his stroke, Sandra talks about the difficulty of convincing her siblings that her father had dementia, that they couldn't be convinced but needed to figure it out for themselves. Or, as Helen adds, "you have to be in it everyday to notice the decline". Other members of the family saw it as a normal part of ageing – "he's getting older, he's starting to get forgetful" – they were in denial about the dementia. They also say that Albert himself was in "denial". This was frustrating because "if somebody could just name this and say something, then at least we can go back and say to the family, 'this is what it is'".

During the conversation we talk about the driving issue, and how it was handled in the November doctor's appointment. It turns out that driving had been a concern for some time previous to this, but one of the reasons Helen hadn't pushed it was because of the two trips they had planned – Helen had wanted to have the holiday "before it's all gone". When she thinks back on it now, she thinks they were "stupid" because of how fast things could happen (that is, Albert's stroke). The issue of driving had also come up in the support group meeting she and Sandra had both attended in August 2015, and was one of the motivators to try to deal with it. When I asked Helen directly if, before their trips last fall, she had a sense that it might be a little "risky" for Albert to be driving, she said no, not really, it "never really registered that way" – she says on the highway he was fine, but he did have trouble finding places. And after the doctor's ban on driving, they also worked out some ways to manage getting to places. Helen would drive – she describes herself as a bad driver, though, as she doesn't know how to park and has tunnel vision – so Albert would do the parking, backing up and so on, and then hand over the keys.

A little later Helen reflects on the experience and what might have been helpful. One of her observations was about not knowing how long – "you'd like to know that somebody could tell you, okay, was he in Stage 1, 2, 3, 4?" It would be helpful because maybe she could adjust a little easier, but then nobody predicted he would have a stroke instead.

Family 3: Ken and Marla Roberts

Ken and Marla were enrolled in the study in August 2015 after Ken received information about the research at an Alzheimer's Society caregiver support group. Marla had been experiencing mild cognitive changes since 2009, mainly related to her memory, that they had both noticed. In 2012 these changes had progressed to a point that Ken wrote a detailed letter to their family doctor describing a gradual reduction in Marla's activities and short-term memory. From this point everyday life became increasingly problematic, with changes in Marla's cognition and behaviour that Ken had some difficulty managing and coping with. Both Marla and Ken became involved with the Alzheimer's Society early on – attending the 'Seeds of Hope' programme, which provides education and support for families in the 'early' stages of dementia. Subsequent sessions deal with middle stage and later stage issues. Ken has attended all of these. He has also done some of his own research for information online, reading scientific articles about the brain and so on.

Ken and Marla's participation in the research was relatively brief but intense. Most field visits involved the formal care system – doctors' visits, day programme observation, attendance at their home when health aides were visiting. By the time of their involvement in the research, Ken was feeling overwhelmed with his day-to-day responsibilities. He had worked it out like this: "we are awake for about 103 hours per week, I have 23 hours of respite, that means 80 hours per week of just me and her and it's like living with a two-year-old." He expressed very firmly that people like him need much more help, and that was his rationale for participating in the research. Marla was admitted to long-term care in October 2015.

Overview

Ken and Marla have been married for almost 50 years. They met in high school. Marla is 69, and Ken is 70. They have two sons. They have no contact with one son, describing the relationship as "estranged", and the other son lives in another city on the other side of the country, although Ken says they have a good relationship, and that he is supportive. Ken speaks with him frequently on the phone and he visits during holidays such as Thanksgiving. They have (or had) what sounds like a fairly wide circle of friends. Ken mentions Marla's "sorority sisters" – long-time women friends who are still in contact but less frequently now and no longer meeting face-to-face (that is, they phone to see how things are). Ken also mentions various neighbours with whom they have friendly relationships. Ken also participates in a men's walking group every Saturday.

Ken is a retired businessman, and was in a management role. Marla worked in retail, women's clothing, until mid-2009, which was when the cognitive problems began to surface – she had difficulty using the computer and till, and was limiting her work activities to hanging clothes, which was not acceptable to her employer. Financially, Ken says he has no concerns about money, and, in fact, he and Marla had planned to spend much of their retirement travelling. They live in a large home in the suburbs – it was custom-built according to their specifications. It is spacious, well furnished, and contains many ornaments on display – although many of these have been moved from their "usual" position because Ken is concerned that Marla will break them, as she has a tendency to "fiddle" and move things around. The house is very tidy, with things apparently having their "proper place". It is notable that one of the clearer comments made by Marla is that "Ken is always fussing". I note this because for the most part her verbal communications are very difficult to make sense of. So it seems possible that Ken is an orderly, managing, even controlling kind of man, and that this has always been part of the dynamic in the family. This also seems apparent in the letters Ken has written to their family doctor and the geriatrician over the past three years – these letters are highly detailed, descriptive accounts of the decline of Marla's abilities and/or behaviours in relation to everyday life, that is, household chores, cooking, dressing, reading, conversational ability, incontinence, and so on. Ken writes these accounts of Marla's condition as part of his preparation for visits to the doctor.

Both Ken and Marla are in good physical condition. Ken is an active member of a walking club, and every week spends some of his respite time with this group. He looks younger than his stated age, and seems to take quite a bit of care with his appearance, also ensuring that Marla is properly groomed – from his comments, this is something that would have been important to her. Marla is also physically well. She is a small woman, thin, but not frail looking. She walks well, and moves about without assistance. She is moving most of the time, wandering about the house.

Marla's cognitive issues seem to have first come to their attention through her work life – she was unable to carry out the tasks necessary to continue her job in retail. Ken also reports gradually seeing her lose the ability to, for instance, use their home computer. He dates this to about mid-2009. It seems that they were able to carry on much as usual, for example travelling and socializing with friends, until early 2012. Throughout the past six years, maintaining their "usual" activities as a couple seems to have been a concern for Ken, for example, continuing their subscription to a dinner theatre even though of late Marla had been unwilling or unable to sit through the event, attending social events such as weddings, going out for dinner, meeting up with her friends, taking short trips to a nearby mountain area and going for walks. Each activity was gradually dropping as Marla's ability to engage or participate declined, or if some event occurred during the occasion that resulted in their needing to leave. For example, Marla "fainted" at a wedding they attended.

It was in May 2014 that the family doctor referred the family to a geriatrician – this seems to have been related to a decline in Marla's MMSE (mini-mental status exam) from 20 to 11 over a period of about nine months. Around this time, several supports were put into place: Marla was enrolled in a day programme for three days per week and home care visited once a week on Saturdays for three hours (so Ken could go out with his walking group). The history of Marla's gradual decline in her abilities is recorded in eight letters Ken wrote to Marla's doctors. In his letters Ken writes about all the things Marla used to do, such as sewing, cooking and entertaining, and that she now had no interest in or ability to continue. His letters end with requests for help to handle the changes that were happening. For example, in his November 2013 letter, he requests an appointment with the family doctor to discuss whether it was safe for Marla to continue driving. In this letter he describes his connection with Marla as 'frail', asking the doctor to take the lead with this discussion about driving. He is also worried at this time about Marla's weight loss and issues with personal hygiene.

Other letters describe his worries about Marla's nutritional status, the risk of infection related to her incontinence, her unwillingness to bathe regularly. Much of Ken's time seems to be taken up with "convincing" Marla to do things – to eat, to bathe. Even seemingly small things, like putting on a coat to go outside, were a struggle – taking time and persuasion and sometimes overriding Marla's objections and unwillingness. By the time I attended the geriatrician's appointment with Ken and Marla in September 2015, Ken was clearly stressed – his note to the doctor details his everyday concerns and frustrations, and notes at the end of the letter, 'I've had to abandon many of my own activities so we spend days locked in our home with nothing to do or even talk about on days when she's not at her day programme'. In this appointment the doctor says she will prioritize placement for Marla.

Placement for Marla happens very quickly after this. The transition coordinator calls Ken the same day as the appointment to begin the process, and two weeks later a bed is found for Marla at a facility that is acceptable to Ken. She is admitted a week later. A few weeks after this I go with Ken to visit Marla. We go for a walk, and sometimes Marla holds Ken's hand. On our return, we stop by her room and put away her outdoor things. Marla wanders off towards the dining room, and when we catch up to her to say goodbye, Ken tries to settle her in to watch some TV. She refuses and seems to want to come with us, but Ken stops a staff member and says he is leaving, and asks if she could take Marla back into the dining room. She does so, and Marla goes with her docilely.

Family 4: Katherine and David Cruz, sons Josh and Brent

Katherine first made contact in August 2015 after hearing about the study at a caregiver support group meeting. She said she was interested but would wait a few months, until January, before the family became actively involved. The Cruz family, Katherine, David and their two sons, were part of the research for one year, from January 2016 until January 2017, when David was admitted to long-term care. Visits included social outings, such as going out for lunch or to a prayer meeting, going along with the family to multiple appointments with doctors, and attendance in their home just for visits or to observe the practices of the home care providers. David is 68, Katherine is 65, and Josh and Brent are both in their early 30s. David and Katherine immigrated to Canada separately many years ago from a Southeast Asian country. They met and married in Canada, and had their family. Both sons currently live at home. Josh is a university student and Brent recently moved back home after being made redundant from his job in another city. The Cruz family live together in a split-level home in a well established, moderate-income neighbourhood in the south part of the city – as the house is split level, this means that it is designed with many stairs – up into the kitchen, down into the family room, and another set up to the second-floor bedrooms.

Overview

Katherine and her sons identify the "problem" as having started about two years ago when Katherine noticed that when she looked at her husband there was something "not there". When David went for his annual physical she mentioned her concerns to the family doctor, who did what sounds like an MMSE and referred them to a geriatrician at the Seniors Clinic. When they went to the clinic, Katherine says that the doctor there said yes, David had dementia. The family say that when David was first diagnosed the impairments were not that obvious – he forgot things here and there, and would forget to pass on messages. At this point, David had been retired from his work as an assembler for about a year, and Katherine had also just retired from her job. While he'd been working, the family hadn't noticed any changes. His initial diagnosis was mild cognitive impairment (MCI); this was recently reclassified as Alzheimer's disease. In their last doctor's appointment, about six months before their involvement in the research, the doctor told them David was 'progressing fast' as measured by a drop in his

MMSE scores. David started taking medication to improve his memory, and to slow down the progress of the disease, but the family hadn't noticed much of a difference.

David has a somewhat complicated health history. As well as the cognitive changes, he is also thought to have Parkinson's disease because he has had several falls that seem related to Parkinson's-like symptoms. He also had hip surgery about a year ago and the family thinks that he may have had a small stroke at that time because something seemed to inhibit his recovery after surgery. He seemed to have persistent weakness on one side, and so has been getting physiotherapy as part of his day programme. Katherine mentions the ability to continue physiotherapy was key to why they chose the day programme David attends – keeping David moving is very important to the whole family.

Sometimes when talking about David Katherine gets a little teary, and says it's been hard because "you can see other people, husbands, they're enjoying their retirement ... here I sit, here I am". Josh suggests that when his father was first diagnosed, there were a few episodes, and he was very independent. He needed some direction, for example, to take his medication, but not much. But as the months have gone by, they are seeing a more general reliance on everyone else, and David needs more and repeated direction. Sometimes they find him lost in the house. He says it is a struggle for them not to say 'you should know this', to recognize it's the disease. So they have a hard time knowing the difference between what he could do and what he will do, and sometimes they see him as stubborn or just unwilling to do things for himself. It started with needing help with his medication, but now it is hygiene, and needing reminding all the time. Josh talks about his dad needing "priming" to complete activities. He can dress himself but only if they lay out his clothes and then remind him lots of times about what to do. Brent, the younger son, echoes these concerns, seeing his father do something one week but then not being able to do it the next. This means there is a lot of friction between Brent and his father – he wants him to do better, so he pushes him – and he sets up rules. Sometimes it works; sometimes it doesn't.

Over the past four months, Josh has noticed his father becoming more hesitant and wanting people with him. Katherine says that Josh describes David as her "shadow".

Because of David's mobility issues – he is currently using a walking frame because of continuing weakness in one leg – and his dislike of being alone, the family has tried to always have someone at home. They check in with each other frequently to adjust schedules, sometimes cancelling planned activities if needed. The doctor has emphasized that

David can't be left home alone. Katherine says "he said it's 24 hours now" – so even at night someone is supposed to be "with" David. But one problem is that David sleeps during the day and is then disruptive at night. He doesn't sleep through the night and bangs the floor with his cane when he wants something. His not sleeping through the night is a problem, albeit one they are getting used to.

Katherine is a busy woman, very engaged in volunteer activities and her prayer group and choir. She and David go together to many of these activities, and most of her friends are pretty good with that – they don't necessarily know what to do, but they "kind of cater to him". David especially likes going where there is food. He doesn't talk much, but Josh says he has always been kind of a quiet person. Brent says it is hard to have a conversation with his father – he doesn't retain anything and will repeatedly ask the same question. One of the biggest frustrations they all mention is that David "doesn't listen", for example, when they give him reasons why he should do his physiotherapy exercises, or not drink too much milk (he also has some swallowing problems). Josh and Katherine have both gone to the Alzheimer's Society support groups – Josh once or twice and Katherine more regularly – but it depends on whether David is willing to go with her (sometimes he says he is tired). Josh says he found the support group frustrating because he had to listen to other people's stories where the person living with dementia was more compliant, and this made him more aware how different their situations were – and trying to compare situations was not helpful. Brent has attended an education session.

Katherine is grateful for her sons' support – because of them, she is able to continue with many of her usual activities. For example, she goes to mass nearly every morning and so Brent helps his father get ready for Katherine to drive him to the day programme when she gets home. Brent also tries to make sure that if he knows his mum has to go out, he will be home – he is home the most. Katherine says because there are three of them, they are able to manage and have not yet needed home care support, although David goes go to a day programme two days a week (even though they are not really sure he enjoys it).

When talking about what helps the most in terms of being able to manage everyday life, Katherine says that they have adjusted to suit David, each one them somewhat differently, but they are all adjusting. And David has also adjusted, easing into new routines and different abilities. Josh describes it like this: "I think he kind of just eased into it. I don't remember him trying to explain himself or minimize a lot of the memory problems. He just kind of went with it." So, as David eased into forgetting, his family eased into reminding and arranging.

Josh adds that it is just having the three of them to work together, and that's probably why David is still able to be at home because they all take turns and fill in the different roles to fill the gaps. Family friends also offer to help some, but not much.

The other challenge is taking David places – needing to think ahead because of accessibility issues, as well as some challenges related to David's behaviour. For example, sometimes he pushes though people with his walking frame on his way to the bathroom. And there are lots of places David needs to go – he has his regular appointments at the Seniors Clinic, appointments with the dentist and the eye doctor, two days a week at the day programme – as well as places they go as a family. All these outings present logistical challenges – parking, getting David's walking frame in and out of the car, if parking is far away, having someone stay with David while the other person parks. In lots of ways, "dementia" is not the biggest problem they are dealing with; rather, a challenge is helping David stay safe, and especially not to fall.

Falling and risk management related to this is a big part of their interactions with health professionals. For example, during visits with the geriatrician, his main concern is David "falling in the house". He has advised them that David must use his walking frame at all times, even in the house, and be supervised 24 hours a day. The doctor says they may need to start thinking about institutional care or 'make changes to his [David's] living situation to make him safe', because his dementia and his falling are linked. But one problem is all the stairs in the house, and Katherine wonders, "maybe we have to rethink the house". In their home David can't really avoid stairs, and he can't use his walking frame on them, and in any case, his most recent fall was in the bedroom where "it was flat". Moving to an apartment, however, would mean that Josh and Brent could no longer live with their parents.

Over the next few months David continues to occasionally fall, mostly in the house as he moves around, or when he gets up to go to the bathroom at night. Most of the falls are "slides" down the wall; he is not injured, but needs help getting back up. Sometimes he gets a cut or a bruise. Once he needed to go to the Emergency Department (A&E) to get stiches. Formal care providers, home care aides and home physiotherapy have become more involved. Cueing and reminding from family to attend to personal hygiene has become less effective, and David is also sometimes incontinent, so home care has workers come in to help David to shower twice a week. Someone now comes in twice a day for morning and evening "grooming". After hearing about one fall at night in the bathroom, David's home physio aide recommends they put a commode by the bedside – but Katherine is not keen on this, as she is not sure how it solves anything.

So there is a bit of a cascade of problems, many of which seem to reference David's (failing) physicality – his falls, the fact that he now he seems to have cataracts, there are dental appointments, there is his incontinence and commode chairs, showers and morning grooming. Although David has a dementia, the household is starting to need to be organized around the care of David's body – it is becoming more difficult to maintain the "norms" of family life. Katherine is now keeping a list of David's falls to share with the doctor, monitoring and accounting for David's "decline". There is a push to find a "safer" place for David to live, and the family is wondering if, given all these concerns, home is still "appropriate". In the next doctor's appointment, falls are again singled out as the most important issue, but some of the things that might help – cataract surgery or more physiotherapy – are not available. The doctor tells them that they are doing their best but that things are going "downhill", and says that a decision may need to be made – "you are doing your best, but it may not be enough".

For the next few months the family is in a bit of a holding pattern, trying to maintain David safely at home, using the home care assistance available to them – they have been told they need to "max out" services before they can even get on a waiting list for placement. Their practices of waiting are active – seeking out and gathering information, interacting with multiple case managers, weighing the pros and cons of various decisions – and all the time trying to meet the "requirement" for 24-hour supervision, a responsibility that has fallen mainly on Brent. But despite everything, Katherine is undecided as to whether an institutional placement would be "better". Eventually, it seems necessary – Katherine is afraid that "something" will happen that they won't be able to handle. Now one of the family always walks beside David, especially up and down the stairs, and even when he "goes to the bathroom, I'm there", Katherine says. David is not getting "better". The assessment form for long-term care placement reads: "difficult for the family to manage … falls, incontinence, feeding". Katherine says she is scared he will fall "and hit his head, especially if I am by myself. What would I do? He hasn't hit his head yet but it seems it is only a matter of time".

David went to live in long-term care in early January 2016. Katherine spent time there with him every day, and I visited with her in late January. By that time he had fallen twice and developed pneumonia. He died in early February 2016.

5

Relations between formal and family care: divergent practices in care at home for people living with dementia

In this chapter we analyse a theoretical and practical problem of longstanding: what are good ways to think about how family care practices and those of the formal system relate? Few would disagree that the ways that families and formal care systems handle daily life are different, with, as noted in Chapter 1, extensive research efforts undertaken over many decades addressing issues that arise from these differences (see, for example, Twigg, 1989; Bond, 1992; Lyons and Zarit, 1999; Zarit et al, 1999; Ward-Griffin and McKeever, 2000; Wiles, 2003; Büscher et al, 2011; Stephan et al, 2018; O'Shea et al, 2019). Yet, despite a long interest in, and study of, relations between family care practices and those of the formal system, difficulties persist, with families reluctant at times to use services that are meant to be helpful or using these supports without experiencing them as helpful.

In this chapter we don't try to 'solve' this problem but rather, we try to understand it differently by following the experiences of the Cruz family, introduced in Chapter 4, and specifically focus on those events in our Field notes that show differences between the family's care practices and those of formal systems. The aim is to consider what, in these specific situations, may be at stake, what types of relations are being enacted and what types of relations might be helpful. This leads us not to 'general rules' stipulating what should be done, or broad claims about how these differing practices should relate, but rather, to a different, more complicated and more located sense of the problem.

As noted previously, the question we are exploring is not a new one, but in this chapter we try to work through it in a new way. To do this we draw on Isabelle Stengers' (2005a, 2005b, 2015 [2009], 2018, 2019) writing about an 'ecology of practices' to theorize the idea of a divergence in family and formal care practices that has implications for care. In Stengers' view, what makes a practice diverge is also what makes it a particular practice; overriding these differences and imposing similarity, such as efforts to 'professionalize' family caregiving, can damage the practice so aligned. In some respects our argument here returns to Bond's (1992) early analysis of the politics of caregiving to examine the 'inherent contradictions' (1992, p 5) in desires to align family and formal care practices chiefly, it seems, through a strategy of 'professionalizing' family carers, for example through education and 'upskilling' (Stajduhar et al, 2010; Sadler and McKevitt, 2013; Ceci et al, 2018a). Note, however, that this is not an argument against offering helpful resources of all sorts to families to assist in their everyday tasks, but rather one that questions what may be at stake when home and the care practised therein begins to be thought, as May (2012, p xii) argues, as no longer a bounded domestic territory but a 'suburb of the health care system itself'. We keep in mind, then, the idea that home is not a 'ready-made' location of healthcare, but becomes actively constituted as such through complex sets of practices that are coordinated by people and by policy instruments. A great deal of work – from people, practices, technologies and organizations – is necessary to constitute and maintain the home as a site of healthcare (Pols, 2012), which suggests there are many and diverse relations to be explored.

While we start with Stengers' ecological framework to argue for an understanding of family and formal care practices as divergent, we also need to think about how such divergent practices might relate. Stengers offers the figure of the diplomat, and the trope of diplomatic relations, to show how diverging practices that have common interests – but not necessarily the same interests in common – could relate in a way that would leave 'borders' and thus practices intact. To this we add texture provided by Law and colleagues (2013) in their discussion of the non-coherence of practices. They, somewhat similarly to Stengers, start from a position that suggests non-coherence among practices is the rule, rather than an exception, but that there are many 'styles of non-coherence' and thus many modes of possible relations (2014, p 175). Again, there is no general rule that tells us how practices relate, but rather working through empirical instances, as we will do in this chapter, may help us to see the ways that coherence is sometimes achieved, albeit partially and temporarily, in a context of non-coherence. Possible relations are discussed by Law and colleagues in terms of modes or styles of syncretism, referring to a range of logics or ordering practices that offer language to talk about different ways of handling non-coherence, where putting practices into words helps us to see how and where practices may fit together, coexist – or not (see also Law, 1994; Moser, 2005; Mol, 2008; Mol et al, 2010). This range of logics, they argue, is always 'at hand', but we need to find ways to think, understand and talk about this (Law et al, 2013, p 174). In their argument, Law et al identify a number of modes or styles of syncretism – not a definitive list, but some good examples for thinking about family and formal care practices. Some examples include denial, where a 'system' can proceed without thinking or caring about the messy processes that make it work (p 178), or 'domestication', where 'non-coherence is recognized but then is domesticated' (p 180). These kinds of ways of relating have relevance, not least because achieving temporary and partial coexistence of divergent practices entails a great deal of work. Making relations that can be lived with is neither easy nor passive (Law et al, 2013). Using these two sets of theoretical resources, in this chapter we try to work through the question of what are good relations between family and formal care practices, and what the goods (and bads) involved may consist of.

As noted previously, our study design involved 'following' families – which meant going along with members of a family on various outings, both 'social' and health-related, as well as spending time with them in their homes, sometimes just visiting and other times observing their interactions with various kinds of formal care providers. On reflection, this study design instituted a certain asymmetry in our data collection, although it could be argued that the design was in some respects set up by the binaries that already exist between formal and family care practices. However, it is also true that our methods in some ways reinscribed these, and we see those effects in our data. So, although we also had interviews with key informants active in the larger context of dementia care (see Chapter 2), it was also the case that we got to know most about the families who were part of the study, what they did, how they thought about things and the kinds of people and structures they encountered. Although we observed the actions of people they met with, for example physicians and nurses, we learned less about how these actors thought about their practices. Our 'nearness' to the participant families is both a clear strength of our design but also one that comes with some limitations: a strength, because we got to see something of what happens when families encounter 'other' practices, and a limitation, as these 'other' practices remain somewhat distal in our analyses insofar as we see what is going on mostly from the position of the families.

With this asymmetry in mind it becomes even more important to avoid what Stengers (2019) describes as the trap of comparing. For example, 'safety' is a big concern in care at home, and in our Field notes a range of differing practices are represented that seem to be about safety, with those of families and those of formal care providers they met with showing important divergence. Certainly for the Cruz family 'safety' issues were of concern from the outset – both for the family and for the formal care providers – but the question of what to do seemed to show divergent repertoires of thinking and action (Mol, 2008). In some respects, it is hard not to see these as being opposed. For example, the Cruz family practices of 'safety' seemed more oriented to the 'real' practicalities of daily life because, in fact, they are and must be; formal care practices that we observed in relation to this family tended to highlight more technical or instrumental issues of risk management. Risk management is a big part of professional practice but carries, and seemed to try to impose, a very different logic of care (Mol, 2008) than that carried by the family's care practices. None of this is surprising, and yet setting these practices in opposition by comparing them is also not particularly helpful – resolution of the observed difficulties becomes a matter of making one practice more 'like' the other, of selecting out good or bad ways to proceed, but always with references to the standards of one or other of the practices. It was coming to this impasse that led us to Stengers' work – if these practices are indeed different, how might we think about the relations between them in a way that avoids the trap of comparison, or at least pays due attention to the ethical and political challenges such comparison entails (Stengers, 2019)? This is an analytical problem, but what makes it worth pursuing is that it is also, as noted previously, a practical one of very longstanding.

Ecology of practices as a 'tool for thinking'

It is in this context that we find the writings of philosopher of science Isabelle Stengers (2005a, 2005b, 2015 [2009], 2018, 2019) about an ecology of practices helpful, even though her main concern is with practices of science. What Stengers offers us is a vocabulary for posing questions about diverging practices, where divergence is understood as constitutive rather than relational. That is, she argues that divergence is what makes a practice a particular practice – but she is careful to emphasize that it is divergence in itself that makes a practice and not divergence from other practices. When we analyse divergence as *divergence from* we fall immediately into the trap of comparison – which is what we are trying to avoid because it always becomes one practice or the other that sets the standard for comparison. Divergence has to do with heterogeneity, and so we need to think about practices as *among* other practices (Savransky and Stengers, 2018).

Stengers' (2005a, 2005b, 2019) ecological vocabulary helps us to make sense of difference without comparing in part because in ecology conflicting interests are 'a general rule' (2019, p 190). Ecology, Stengers suggests, 'has no point of contact with the ideal of peace, harmony or good will (in which all parties are asked to bow down to some general interest)' (2019, p 188). Neutrality or a neutral point of view is not an option, and since no practice can be comfortably defined as just 'like any other', we must stay with the idea of contrast, difference and divergence among practices, and eventually with a question of how divergent practices relate. Stengers (2005a, p 185) offers ecology of practices as a 'tool for thinking through what is happening' – it is not a structure that somehow enables the representation of practices as they 'really are' but rather, it is a way to make more likely the asking of pertinent questions about divergence and less likely the explaining away of difference. Thus as a tool, working with the idea of an ecology of practices helps to 'reset' usual understandings of possible relations between family and formal care practices in part through 'the construction of new "practical identities" for practices, that is, new possibilities for them to be present, or in other words to connect' (Stengers, 2005a, p 186). Part of this reset involves regarding both sets of protagonists as practitioners despite the ambiguity introduced by this move. Rather than pre-designate some involved as, for example, users or consumers, and others as providers, and thus embed assumptions about both problem and solution, all are regarded as 'bearers of recognized knowledge', contributing to a common concern but not defining it (Stengers, 2015 [2009], p 88).

Divergent practices

Beginning with what Stengers (2019) herself describes as an unusual understanding of practices helps to avoid easy familiarity: the term 'practice' denotes 'any form of life that is bound to be destroyed by the imperative of comparison and the imposition of a standard ensuring equivalency, because what makes each one exist is also what makes it diverge' (2019, p 187). This is an understanding of practices that seems to have more at stake than most, underscoring both the positivity of divergence and the possibility of destruction – in an ecology, struggles are for existence. As Stengers (2018, p 87) writes, the concept of practices she introduces is 'not meant to be a peaceful one'. Divergence here refers to the ways in which a practice has 'its own positive and distinct way of paying due attention; that is, of having things and situations matter. Each produces its own line of divergence, as it likewise produces itself' (Stengers, 2019, p 187). When these lines of divergence are overcome, the practice, as a particular practice, is destroyed. Positively, divergence, as found in an ecology, helps to define 'relational heterogeneity' (2019, p 187), pointing to a plurality that can exist when one is not folded into the other. One situation in ecology that Stengers references in this respect is symbiosis: 'symbiosis meant that these beings are related by common interests, but common does not mean having the same interests in common, only that diverging interests now need each other' to achieve their own pathways and goals (2019, p 188). There can be a relation, or many kinds of relations, but to survive each practice must retain its 'full force', continuing to diverge and define in its own terms what matters, able to resist the impositions of the other (2019, p 190).

Comparison, which we have referred to previously, is one process by which impositions may be forced and a practice may be weakened. In order to compare, a commensurability must be instituted between practices, to align the practices, to impose similarity or to normatively demonstrate better or worse ways to proceed, a process that is never neutral but rather relative to the aim of the comparison. That is, comparison happens with reference to a standard, goal or other criteria that may or may not be relevant in the context of the divergent practices at issue. Worse case is when comparison is conducted unilaterally, 'in the language of just one of the parties' (Stengers, 2019, p 184). This is not a good situation, one that in an ecology is akin to a predator/ prey relation: 'practices that maintain stronger definitions will freely define others as prey' (2019, p 187). Of course, as Stengers argues, it is the imperative of comparison rather than comparison itself that makes the problem: 'the imperative always means the imposition of a standard that presupposes and enacts silence, the impossibility of objecting or of demanding due attention' (2019, p 186).

Approaching a practice, suggests Stengers (2005a, p 184), 'means approaching it as it diverges, that is, feeling its borders'. This is the intent of the ethnographic descriptions we now turn to: feeling the borders, being concerned with differences in how a family handles daily life and the ways those borders become visible in interactions with the 'outside'. Few would disagree that there are differences between family care practices and professional care practices even when the practices at issue may share common interests, and indeed, may need each other. But even though difference is often recognized, it seems easily explained away through appeals to common goals. As noted previously, in this chapter we focus our discussion on 'safety' as one such common goal. Safety, in its diverse manifestations, is important for the social and policy goal of keeping people living with dementia at home for as long as possible: adverse events of various kinds precipitate crises and create a requirement for action from formal systems, which is something everyone seems to want to avoid. So safety is a problem for daily life and for formal care systems – there is a common interest – but, as Stengers (2019) argues, common does not mean that diverging practices have the *same* interests in common.

Feeling borders: stories about 'safety'

We have put safety in scare quotes in our heading here because we are not certain that safety is exactly what these stories are 'about'. It might be better to simply describe the stories as showing different ways of handling the practicalities of daily life. At the same time, safety is a recognizable way to talk about different practices of care at home, becoming so important in academic practice, for example, that some describe it as a 'new research frontier' (MacDonald et al, 2013, p 126). And developing knowledge about 'safety' through research is one approach to 'improving' care at home as well as influencing the nature of safe professional home care practice. These are important efforts and much work has been undertaken to learn about risk factors, risk profiles, system weaknesses and interventions that might support families to be better able to manage identified risks and thus support the larger policy goal of delaying institutionalization (see, for example, CPSI, 2013; Lach and Chang, 2007; Afram et al, 2014; Stevenson et al, 2018). Knowledge about risks and how to 'best' handle them are significant elements of professional practices, something to which informed practitioners will pay due attention; it is part of what makes their practices professional or 'knowledge/evidence-based'. As Stengers (2015 [2009], p 90) writes, 'the knowledge of a practitioner, her capacity to participate in the construction of a problem, refers to the community to which she belongs'. We could say that discourses of risk management 'belong' to professional healthcare practice, and practitioners have obligations in terms of these to which they are accountable (Stengers, 2005a). That is, practitioners are not universally obligated but are obligated in terms of those attachments that make their practice, that show what matters to the practice and what the practice itself demands.

Practices of 'paying due attention': the Cruz family

The Cruz family, whose story we highlight in this chapter, had their 'own positive and distinct way of paying due attention' (Stengers, 2019, p 188) to matters that could be said to be 'about' safety. However, it could not be said that they are attached to discourses of risk management in the same way as professional practitioners. As described in Chapter 4, this family is made up of Katherine and David Cruz, and their two adult sons Brent and Josh, both of whom live in the family home with their parents. David has a complicated health history. Alongside 'memory problems' that had increased over the past two years and a diagnosis of dementia six months prior to the first author's involvement (Christine Ceci), there was history of a Parkinson's-type illness that affected his mobility. David's Parkinson's-like symptoms had made walking difficult and he had already experienced several falls related to 'foot drop'. So, along with concerns about altered cognition, David's falls were a problem that needed to be looked after. Our first excerpt from the Field notes shows one way in which this was done, the practical handling of 'safety' in the day-to-day life of the family. Although this description of going out for lunch offers only a glimpse of daily practices, it does show something of the family 'ethos', which Stengers (2019, p 187) would describe as the specific terms through which their 'needs, behaviours, habits and crucial concerns' positively diverge in producing the family practice and, because this is an ecological framing, in meeting their specific environment:

FIELD NOTES

March 2016

We put our coats on and start to walk down the street to the cafe. Josh has gone to get the car and move it closer to the cafe. David is pushing his walker [walking frame], and I become aware of just how uneven the sidewalk [pavement] is as he seems to catch one of the sliders on every crack. It's about a half a block of slow walking to the intersection, and then we cross at the crosswalk [pedestrian crossing]. The sidewalk is cut for accessibility but it is still a little slow for us to get across the intersection. Inside the cafe we find a table, David says loudly he is hungry, and Katherine and I help him get settled in a chair. Josh comes in and they discuss what to eat, and what to get for David to eat. Katherine and I order coffee and sit back down with David; in minutes Josh is putting a plate of pasta in front of his dad. He also orders a sandwich for them to share. Then David says he has to go to the bathroom and Josh goes off to find the location. He comes back and gets his dad.

Slowing down to observe, but still recognizing that the intricacies of daily practices are hard to put into words (Mol, 2008), we can see the people, objects and relations involved in the practice; we start to see to what the family is 'paying due attention'. The family's practice clearly includes 'considerations of safety' but points to something else that is more complex (Winthereik and Verran, 2012). The walk outside shows the materials and relations that are part of the family's arrangements: the car being moved, the walking frame being moved over the uneven pavement, David's slow and careful steps and those walking with him matching their pace with his, the timing of the pedestrian crossing, the restaurant tables and the accessibility of the bathroom. The family, as a collective that obviously includes David, works to navigate the space in what seems a precarious way – the fit is not quite good between the pavement and the walking frame, bathroom access has to be scoped out. 'Safety', we could say, emerges through these moment-to-moment embodied practices of navigating the logistics of the outing, accommodating the body and behaviour of David, making up for the mismatch between the space and time of the world outside their home and their ability to be in it.

The ethos of the family care practice here involves this specific responsiveness to each other, to David's current abilities, to the goal of the outing and its locale. There are some 'risks' here as well, but they have a place as practical 'here-and-now' problems of *this* family accomplishing *this* activity, not the universal ones of preventing falls for people-like-David who have cognitive issues and foot drop (Stengers, 2019). The singularity shows what matters here and not somewhere else, a distinction that signals a border, as well as what Mol (2008) describes as a 'whole world' showing its specific, embedded logic: the specific ways in which the family organizes their actions and interactions, the ways David moves his body and Katherine and Josh support this, how they know each other and anticipate needs. Each part of the practice shows what the people involved, or, in Stengers' (2005a, p 191) terms, the practitioners, are attached to, with attachments being 'what causes people to feel and think, to be able or become able'. The achievement of the outing is not an achievement of a general sort, but of the family as belonging to this practice, obliged and exposed by their attachments – to each other and to these specific circumstances (Stengers, 2005a, p 192). And at the risk of having this one story carry too much weight, we would argue that this relational ethos, tied to a specific context, shows something of the family care practice in its 'full force', defining in its own terms what matters (Stengers, 2019, p 184). To maintain the borders of the practice we should not, as Stengers (2005a, p 193) argues, apply or insist on an 'extra-territorial' way of defining what matters here by, for example, suggesting that the careful movements through the street are, or even are 'like', the professional practice of risk management. Although different kinds of 'risk' are undoubtedly carefully being 'managed' here, the practice does not rely on deliberative strategies of assessment or mitigation. Rather, the family practice is moved by a logic of contingency, responsive to what is happening in the moment with the materials at hand (Law et al, 2013), with 'care' and carefulness distributed across the multiple actors – material and human – involved (Schillmeier, 2017). They are being careful in specific located ways through a knowledgeable practice that suits them and no one else simply because it is characteristic of their specific attachments and their ways of handling the 'unfolding uncertainties' of their daily life (Law et al, 2013 p 183). This is the first feature to keep in mind – there is a coherence in this practice that is knitted together in good ways to accomplish what matters to the practitioners. As Moser (2011, p 714) would say, this is a 'relational ordering' – life is being in relation, which also 'implies being *held* in connection, being *made* part of, and so sharing in, a collective and the practices that carry it' (original emphasis). Our question, then, is what kinds of relations are instituted when this family care practice encounters practices that are located 'outside' their borders, practices that may be animated by a different logic?

Practices of 'paying due attention': the logics of formal care

When we think about the idea of formal care practices as being 'outside' family care practices, it may be helpful to think about the logics that inform some of these activities and the differences that make them divergent practices. To stay true to Stengers' analysis, we try to do this without positioning these as divergent *from* family practices. The idea here is that if a practice is constituted through the matters to which it pays due attention, as well as its specific ways of paying due attention, then there will be, as Nocek (2018, p 99) argues, differences in practices that cannot be either simply explained away or accounted for in advance. Before showing what we mean with some examples from the Field notes, it is important to note that we are not suggesting that there are not a lot of challenges for families that come along with a diagnosis of dementia, including challenges that formal care practices can help with. There is significant research examining these, trying to address all those concerns that arise from the need to tend to the practicalities of daily life and care that is enacted in a restricted space (the home) over a prolonged period of time, and concerning a person who may require almost constant attention (Askham et al, 2007). Both families and formal care providers are very attuned to these – but we want to argue this attunement is something that takes different forms, even when the practitioners involved share a concern such as safety.

A good example of this from our Cruz family Field notes is an idea that appears repeatedly – that David, to be kept safe, which generally seems to mean to be prevented from falling, requires 24-hour supervision. In the initial family interview at the start of the fieldwork, Katherine shared that "the doctor, according to the senior doctor, he said it's 24 hours. When he said that he's even worse [that is, that David was showing signs of increasing cognitive decline], he said it's 24 hours now so we don't leave him" (family interview, January 2016). In a subsequent clinic visit, the nurse conducting the initial assessments started her interview with David and Josh by inquiring 'about how David is doing at home, and if the family is "supervising him 24 hours"' (Field notes, January 2016). Later, during this same appointment, the doctor also draws attention to the kind of care David is seen to require:

FIELD NOTES
January 2016

The doctor now turns attention to David's mobility, asks whether or not he is using his walker [walking frame] at home, in the house? The family is non-committal about this, start to say that it is difficult to use the walker inside. The doctor asks about a cane, especially for going up and down stairs. David says he uses it 'always'. Doctor reiterates his primary concern is falls. The doctor then turns to Katherine and Brent and Josh, and says that David may need more care 'down the road', and now may be time to start that. ... At this point he says again, 'safety is most important – if the home is not safe, despite the changes made ... you need to make changes to his living situation to make him safe, changes in lifestyle, maybe a different apartment or assisted living.' 'David must use his walker all the time.' ... The doctor then adds, 'in spite of all the things you may do, events happen, David needs 24-hour supervision – safety is most important.'

Twenty-four-hour supervision, a practice that is concerned with surveillance and monitoring, has a long institutional history. For health professionals, such supervision is often seen as legitimate and necessary, and is performed across diverse, although mainly institutional, settings. It is an existent practice that assumes presence in the form of observation and proximity will contribute to safety, or at least help to assure desired outcomes – in David's case, this would be fewer or no falls. It is a practice oriented to controlling future events and in some kinds of institutional settings, this practice has a specific sense and meaning – although it must be noted that even in institutional care, it is still not, except in exceptional circumstances, practised literally as constant observation of a person over 24-hour periods of time. Yet a practice informed by an institutional-surveillance logic, one that is rarely performed even in institutions, is repeatedly – over time and across multiple formal care actors – proposed as necessary for David and his family.

What makes this situation worth exploring in terms of the non-coherence of practices is that there is a lot at stake for everyone involved. For health system practices there is the 'good' of offering expert advice, maintaining positioning as the trusted source of such advice, and the more specific possibility of keeping David from being injured in a fall, thus avoiding the need for more professional care. What makes the logic of surveillance hard to argue with is that David does fall, and having someone with him at all times would likely go some way to prevent this. And it may not be that the Cruz family *must* incorporate institution-like practices into their home life but there seems to be 'risks' in not working in this direction: a custodial practice of ensuring safety is offered as a possible future, and associated with the conditions in which David may continue to reside in his home: "if the home is not safe. ..." The risk of losing David is a bad to be avoided. So it would seem that interests are aligned and everything fits, but only if all the 'messy differences' in family and formal care practices are ignored, and only if the family practice changes to take on more institution-like arrangements (Law et al, 2013, p 173). Notably, the Cruz family's practices of knowing, acting and understanding both David and the character of their daily lives, as well as David's own propensities to act in ways that reflect his own wishes, become muted in this context.

How do these differences get smoothed over in the clinic setting? To begin, in determining the need for a practice such as surveillance, expert knowledge figures prominently. For Stengers (2005b, p 1000), experts 'are the ones whose practice is not threatened by the issue under discussion since what they know is accepted as relevant'. They present themselves and what they know 'in a mode that does not foresee the way in which that knowledge will be taken into account' (Stengers, 2005b, p 1000). For David, the case for 24-hour supervision is built up through a range of careful standardized clinical assessment practices that work to relate his current medical situation with known risk factors, as well as the nature of known, useful prevention strategies. Although David and his family are enrolled in the process of information gathering and questions are asked about how they are managing, this practice also follows a clear clinical protocol about what is important to know. Nobody involved questions this, which brings to mind Stengers' (2019, p 186) caution that a risk to a practice can be brought about when standards are imposed that include the 'impossibility of objecting'. For example, when the doctor suggests the family may need to rethink their home, it seems to be presented as standard advice, and no one offers information about whether this is possible in their specific circumstances. Similarly, the advice that David requires 24-hour supervision is not challenged. Both instructions contain a general or universal kind of logic, and although the doctor's words do not exactly assume safety is one thing, the framing of the 'solutions' suggests that 'these' actions would somehow work for everyone. For this practice, for someone 'like' David who forgets and falls, a home without stairs and 24-hour supervision is insurance against bad things happening.

In one sense the relation between these practices is one of denial of non-coherence (Law et al, 2013) insofar as in the appointment nobody actually acknowledges a lack of fit between the logic of the care practised by the family, one that depends on what is happening and the materials at hand, and that of maintaining a practice of sustained observation and surveillance. The willingness of everyone to go along – David, his family, the nurse, the doctor – reflects a practically embedded knowledge about how things are usually done in this location where expert advice is offered, usually assumed to be relevant and without too much worry to establish how that knowledge will be taken into account (Stengers, 2005b). It is also probably important for the family not to acknowledge the possibility of failing to deliver the desired outcome, as to do so might imply that they lack the necessary resources – knowledge, care and material – to ensure David's safety. They might appear incompetent, and there is pressure to avoid giving this sort of impression. That is, the location itself, and the extent to which it represents a 'system' that the Cruz family may not need now but will likely need down the road, frames what will count as a good way to handle difference (Law et al, 2013). In other words, it is a good for everyone to not point out the lack of fit. The 'bad', of course, is the extent to which "the system" imposes, or seeks to impose, a single version of the good (Law et al, 2013, p 191) – as well as the amount of work the Cruz family may have to undertake to maintain their 'borders'.

The question for the Cruz family, and for us, is what kinds of relations can be made with this apparently necessary 'border' incursion. In the clinic, non-coherence can be denied, partly because practices can be kept separate. The messiness of everyday life can be imagined here, but is simply not visible.

When divergent practices need each other

Part of what we need to think about is that if the logic of risk management, for example, is drawn into the home, something 'new' is being asked of families, and their practices are being reshaped; they need to make new relations. It could be argued that families would be better off if their practices were more like those of formal care practices, which seems to be part of a powerful dynamic of 'professionalizing' family carers that relies on an assumption of a common interest that is the same interest. Yet this doesn't account for the ways the Cruz family's care practices are constrained in advance by that to which they are attached or the work it will take to make these forms of practice co-exist, to make at least a partial connection, and, perhaps most importantly, the costs or risks for families when even such partial connections start to fray.

Since the family has been advised that David needs 24-hour supervision, they have responded by rotating this role, they talk, they compromise and change their plans, they take turns – practices that work to maintain the family as a family rather than a 'group of caregivers' – but still respond or relate to the formal care practice of supervision. Brent describes it this way 'we just do our stuff [Laughter]. If he needs help, then we're there' (family interview, January 2016). In essence they form a relation to the practice of 24-hour supervision that domesticates it, turns it into something that coheres after all and at least for a while (Law et al, 2013, p 178). This is a good because the trade-offs they make help David stay safe and keep their practices intact: the risks he faces are enacted as something 'real' but also contextual, relative to family relations, material circumstances and even the exigencies of daily life. This is not exactly a practice of 24-hour supervision, but rarely is David left alone. This is a family that lives together, helps each other, but they also have their own activities. But in the course of all of this, David still sometimes falls:

FIELD NOTES

January 2016

Katherine says 'Dr K says we have to have a walker [walking frame] in the house'. The problem is that the house is not really set up for a walker – it is a split-level style, so there is a short flight of stairs from the front hall to the kitchen, and then another short flight from the kitchen down to the family room, and then a longer flight of stairs up to the bedrooms. It is practically impossible to avoid stairs and still have some use of the house. Katherine says, 'maybe we have to rethink the house' meaning maybe they have to think about relocating, probably just she and David (and not the two sons), to an apartment without stairs.

Location creates a concrete and specific problem – a home for a family becomes a location of risk when viewed through a lens of 'risk management'. Home is now something that may need to be rethought, something that is causing trouble.

FIELD NOTES

January 2016

In the hallway, Katherine and Brent talk to me about the doctor's concerns about falls. Katherine says that in their home, David can't avoid stairs, and he can't use a walker [walking frame] for them, and besides that David's most recent fall was in the bedroom where it was 'flat'. How can he avoid stairs in our house, she asks.

Despite the doctor's, and the family's, concerns, the home is not something easily domesticated – although changes can be made in terms of materials such as safety rails and practices such as walking alongside David (especially on the stairs), it is simply not very accommodating of David's walking frame. There are real risks of falling in the relations between the physical space and David and David's walking frame. In this setting there is a conflict between risk management protocols and keeping the family together, an impossible mix of goods and bads to be dealt with: 'I ask Katherine how she thinks she would manage if she did not have her sons living with her – she seems at a loss, and says finally "I couldn't, I could not do it"' (Field notes, May 2016). The Cruz family is sensitive to this non-coherence, that not everything can be fixed:

FIELD NOTES

November 2016

Josh says 'he [David] is falling quite a lot' and describes one morning needing to take his mom to the bus stop and 'when I came home, he was on the floor.' Katherine adds she needed a ride because she was late. I ask if they are worried and Josh says 'so far nothing broken'.... I ask what else might help them and Katherine says 'what else is there?' and shakes her head saying 'I don't know.'

In their day-to-day life they are with David but not necessarily supervising him; sometimes they are sleeping; at other times they need unexpectedly to dash out to the bus stop. A problem, then, is how to associate these divergent practices. If the practices are compared, a new risk arises: formal care assumptions about the problem and how it should be dealt with may end up enacting the family, whose care practices diverge, as failing. As Katherine says later about David continuing to fall, 'we're bad' (Field notes, November 2016). David continuing to fall is not irrelevant to the family, but there is a tension between the confidence that identified strategies will help and how the family handles day-to-day life.

It is at this point an essential asymmetry of relations among practices (Stengers, 2018) becomes more visible, and the ways in which the Cruz family will no longer be able to 'go on in defining in their own manner what matters for them' become clearer (Stengers 2019, p 187). The sense of Katherine's 'we're bad' signals a shift away from the previous looseness of the family's care practices, and the seeming need now to incorporate or relate in a new way to a new logic, to become more clinical: 'Katherine has been holding a notebook with the pages open, I can see it has a list of dates – she is now keeping track of his falls and "incidents"' (Field notes, November 2016).

More objects are being added into care – the suggestion of a commode by the bedside, a notebook tracking falls, and more interventions including daily hygiene assistance for David. Family relations shift to this more clinical mode, making David now, at least for part of the time, an 'object' to observe and track, a body to be taken care of. Some part of this is related to the nature of dementia, a condition in which cognitive and physical abilities decline over time. For everyone involved, the precarities of David's body are increasingly difficult to live with – how to handle this? New equipment, new problems enact new values and relations, creating both 'bridges' and tensions, and when it becomes hard to keep the logics of the two worlds separate, even creating a bit of conflict. The differences between family and formal care practices are increasingly flattened out. The goal in an ecology of practices would be to enable both practices to diverge, that is, to 'go on in defining in their own manner what matters for them' (Stengers, 2019, p 187), but for the Cruz family, it seems their usual ways of handling daily life become overwhelmed.

In some respects there almost seems an inevitability to these border incursions, the family needs the formal care system to carry on day to day, and the formal care system needs these 'family caregivers' to stay actively involved in shouldering the day-to-day work of caring for David. In an ecology this holds the potential to be the 'symbiosis' referred to earlier, a way in which practices remain intact but relate because they need each other to accomplish their own goals – but in this specific case, we still have to understand Katherine's sense of failure contained in her words, "we're bad". So another way to understand what is happening with the Cruz family practices is what Stengers (2018, p 86), referencing Bruno Latour, describes as the difference between relations of peace and those of pacification; peace implies 'fit' with other worlds, pacification implies 'capture' (see also Savransky and Stengers, 2018). In an email a few weeks later Katherine writes:

FIELD NOTES

December 2016

I talked it over with Josh and Brent, and also with friends, they were able to convince me that David will be better in the long-term care rather at home since he is not going to get better but it will be in the worst situation. His right leg is getting harder every day. I will be calling home care OT [occupational therapy] for a wheel chair .... We tried our best to keep him at home, we have our frustration, sometimes angry since for whatever we do David is not getting well and his coughing is getting worst due to his swallowing problem. Are we burned out by all this?

The anticipation of decline and fear of new crises shift how the family sees the fit of home for David, and Katherine's words read like a surrender; they have fought the good fight and just can't do it anymore.

The case for diplomacy

In the beginning we suggested, and have tried to show through this chapter, that family care practices and formal care practices are divergent, that each is characterized by its own distinct way of paying due attention to what matters, with distinct needs, behaviours and crucial concerns. We have tried to show something about what this may look like from the perspective of what we observed of the Cruz family practices, as these shifted to accommodate new relations with 'outside' practices that they now needed. But at the same time, there was also work to keep family practices intact, continuing concern for maintaining and caring for their arrangements, attachments and obligations to each other and their shared way of living. It is this that makes the metaphor of borders so crucial, when encounters with an 'outside' have effects for these relations, or even undo them.

We know the story we've told could be criticized as one-sided, and that we have focused on one thing – concern with safety – showing little of other crucial concerns that may be animating formal care practices or the specific relations practitioners may have tried to make with the Cruz family from the perspective of these practitioners. But this would be missing the point. Our main concern was to try to think through family care practices in a new way, one that began from an assumption of divergence and in so doing, contribute to building a new 'practical identity' for these practices that would, in turn, help us to find new ways to connect (Stengers, 2019).

In thinking through what families are doing as they seek and accept help from the formal care system, the amount of work done by the Cruz family was striking to us, both to sustain borders but also to make new relations, requiring acts of translation and adjustment within their own practice and with outside practices that they now needed. The Cruz family met the non-coherence among these practices in a number of ways: handling difference by denying it, keeping non-coherent practices separate or domesticating what was seen as necessary but still didn't really fit. But also striking was the asymmetry of these relations, especially the extent to which adjustment seemed always underwritten in the language of formal care practices, with the Cruz family holding much, if not all, the responsibility for work at the borders.

There is a sense in which the formal care system and its practices can proceed oblivious of borders. For example, the formal instructions given to the Cruz family show the ways that 'safe' care at home is already imagined to rely on institution-like practices revealing the extent to which, in imagination at least, their home is already pre-figured as an extension of the healthcare system. It is this asymmetry of relations that raises a question of to what extent can a 'system' – powerful, expert, seemingly solidly patterned – actually fit with other worlds rather than capturing them (Stengers, 2018)? This makes a difficult task for formal care practitioners interested in changing the conditions for engaging with families.

New practices of engaging with families is where Stengers' (2005a, 2005b, 2019) figure of the diplomat becomes relevant. In an interview with Martin Savransky, Stengers describes diplomats as 'those who do not address humans in general, but humans as attached, as diverging' (Savransky and Stengers, 2018, p 141). The diplomat will never say 'why don't you just agree' to what I am proposing because diplomatic relations begin with knowledge of humans as 'constrained by diverging attachments' (Stengers, 2005a, p 193). The challenge, suggests Stengers, 'is not to cross the boundary, not to overcome boundaries, but given the boundary, to explore what could be exchanged' (Savransky and Stengers, 2018, p 142). In diplomatic relations, borders between family and formal care practices may become zones of exchange but, as in diplomatic relations between countries, there is no general opening of borders. This is the first point, thinking practices *among* other practices.

However, and perhaps unexpectedly, in Stengers' (2005a, p 193) analysis, diplomacy is not a matter of negotiation or goodwill, a stance that may disrupt those of us who are accustomed to thinking that negotiating relations between formal and family practices would be a good thing. For Stengers, negotiation requires borders to shift to assure common interests, and we want the borders of divergent practices to remain intact. The goal is to achieve peaceful, albeit partial and temporary coexistence, and to avoid pacification. This starts, suggests Stengers, by opening the question of 'what is proper to each practice. Rather than to claim [each] as a practice *like* any other' (Savransky and Stengers, 2018, p 137, emphasis in original). Relating with borders intact, it becomes more possible we will see that the problem a family may be having is not a 'universal problem mattering to everybody' (Stengers, 2005a, p 193), but a problem where 'the specificity and proximity of connections matter' (van Dooren, 2014, cited in Haraway, 2016, p 173). Located and locatable, problems arise in the here and now of *this* family and other practitioners, including formal carers, may be able to help. Stengers suggests a stance of 'experimental togetherness' (2005a, p 195) – local, pragmatic articulations among practices that rely on partial connections among practitioners who are constrained by, but also addressed through, diverging attachments. Rather than eradicating the diverging, practical attachments that make a practice a particular practice, such partial connections are fostered through attention to learning what works and how, as well as when and for whom – not in a general way, but in terms of distinct practices meeting one another in their 'full force'.

6

Patterning dementia

In Chapter 5 we started a process of thinking through divergent practices, those of families and formal care providers, as well as some of the kinds of relations family practices must make with 'other' practices. In thinking through this question of relations between practices, it is impossible not to see, and discuss, the effects of the 'patterning' of dementia in family practices. In this chapter we focus more specifically on this idea of patterning, exploring how each family needed to make relations with the dominant dementia discourse – specifically, the changes each needed to make to remain 'in sync' with the idea of the 'dementia trajectory'.

As has been well established in multiple disciplines, medicine serves a powerful organizing function in people's experiences of health and illness (see, for example, Armstrong, 1982; Gubrium, 1986; Cohen, 1998; Dillman, 2000; Beard, 2016), with the biomedical gaze an exemplar of a way of seeing that looks for patterns, that systematizes in order to know and to intervene (Foucault, 2003). Identifying and ordering 'disorder' through the concept of disease, biomedical discourses and practices also direct how such disorder should be perceived and acted on (Dillman, 2000; Holstein, 2000). An important element of this influence is, as Foucault points out, the anteriority of the medical gaze: 'one now sees the visible only because one knows the language' (2003, p 140). The analytical structure, he suggests, precedes the picture, providing knowledge 'not of what "is" but of the anteriority of ordering' (2003, p 140). Thus the perceived '"givenness" of the disease model' itself (Holstein, 2000, p 171), its easy recognition and mostly smooth application, becomes important in our current context where Alzheimer's disease and other dementias have become the dominant medicalization of old age (Cohen, 1998; Lock, 2013; Latimer, 2018), and where the phenomenon of ageing itself has become deeply associated with a 'crisis rhetoric' (Beard, 2016, p 5). As discussed in previous chapters, fears of demographic ageing, connected explicitly to predictions of an increasing incidence of dementia and the grave threats this is thought to pose to the future sustainability of health and social care systems, mobilize research and policy and shape public attitudes and knowledge (Holstein, 2000; Lock, 2013; Latimer, 2018). As Latimer argues, discourses of crisis and 'epidemic' (see also Lock, 2013) consolidate the medicalized 'ageing–dementia relation' with dementia coming to 'personify all that is most feared about growing old' (2018, p 833).

Magnifying the problematics of this context is the ready availability of 'dementia' discourses that call on us to be 'concerned' and on the look-out for signs of this 'dread' disease in ourselves or in our loved ones (Gubrium, 1986). In the more than three decades since Gubrium's analysis of the public culture associated with Alzheimer's disease, signs and symptoms of dementia, its 'trajectory' and consequences for caregivers have become entrenched as part of our stock knowledge (Schutz, 1946), offering a substantive, and substantially medicalized, vocabulary for making sense of possible experiences we may have in growing old. Although there are ongoing controversies and debates in the scientific literature, including disagreements about the relationship of 'normal' age-related change to that which can be construed as pathological, or in clarifying the etiology, effective treatment and course of a dementia in those so diagnosed (Gubrium, 1986; Whitehouse and George, 2008; Lock, 2013; Haaksma et al, 2019), the public discourse is much smoother. For example, the information found on most Alzheimer Society websites across diverse nations (see, for example, in Canada, https://alzheimer. ca/en/Home or in India, www.alz.org/in/dementia-alzheimers-en.asp) offers substantially the same 'general facts' about dementia, describing a predictable pattern of gradual onset, and progression through stages, culminating in total dependence on the care and supervision of others. This patterning sets out 'progression' within a time frame, or a dementia trajectory, and websites are likely to link this trajectory with the need for advance planning while offering tips and tools to track and manage this progression. In one case, site users are offered the opportunity to calculate 'Alzheimer life expectancy' based on their 'loved one's' performance on an MMSE and the family caregiver's assessment of other 'symptoms' (Dementia Care Central, nd). Dementia awareness campaigns and training programmes work alongside such information providing web resources, pushing to improve 'dementia literacy', urging everyone to 'know the signs, help those who are affected and get vital information on this disorder' (see, for example, Open Learn, nd). It is the apparent power of this patterning of dementia, its scale and scope, which underlines the importance of posing questions about patterning, to the extent that these ways of thinking dementia work to constitute the conceptual space through which people make sense of their experiences of cognitive change and/or 'memory troubles', especially as they age (see also Beard and Fox, 2008; Peel, 2014).

Our aim in this chapter is not so much to debate whether this biomedical patterning of dementia, in particular the 'trajectory discourse', is 'good' or 'bad', accurate or not, but rather to consider what this particular patterning brings for the families involved with our research. What does it lead to? How is it helpful and what does it help with? And, perhaps most interestingly, how does it fit, or not fit, with the ways these families handle daily life in the context of dementia? This last question is important because while there was 'patterning' evident in all of our data, it was also the case that each family was kind of 'like' the pattern, but also kind of not like the pattern. While this variability could be explained with reference to a separation between 'the disease' that stays the same and has similar effects for 'everyone' versus experiences of the disease that are allowed to differ from person to person (Gubrium, 1986; Dillman, 2000; Mol, 2002), we sidestep this opposition by asking instead, how are these related? That is, how do assumptions about the nature of the problem – what it is and what should or can be done about it – contribute to the ongoing shape of care?

As we started to show in Chapter 5, we start from a view that families already have their own relations and deeply historical ways of patterning daily life, and that in the actual practice of daily living there is an inevitable mixing of events, processes, relations and resources that means that, in the end, each family handles daily life, 'does' dementia, differently. But alongside the diverse 'pre-diagnosis' circumstances and practices of families, there is also a biomedical patterning of dementia that is powerful, particularly in its capacity to homogenize experience (Gubrium, 1986), but also to structure and direct experience along some lines and not others. Biomedical patterning of dementia, then, is what Star (1990) describes as a standardizing technology. Her interest, as is ours in this chapter, is in examining the interactions between the stabilizing and homogenizing effects of a powerful practice such as biomedicine and the practices of people who inhabit multiple (other) social worlds, or more to the point, live in 'many worlds at once' (Star, 1990, p 30). A problem we explore, then, is that of 'standards' and the processes of 'translating the images and concerns of one world into that of another' (Star, 1990, p 32). So, while the biomedical patterning of dementia is influential, this influence also needs to be understood against the diverse ways that families do the work of using patterns, including the biomedical. 'Encounters with standards', writes Star, are complexly woven and indeterminate', having to do with multiplicity, partial commitments and partial connections (1990, p 50).

To understand this better, in this chapter we describe family arrangements as they shift and change in navigating and negotiating the conceptual space afforded by the converging discourses of 'the dementia trajectory'. Different enactments (Mol, 2002) of dementia can be seen as outcomes of this inevitable mixing of biomedical discourses that work to pattern ageing and dementia in particular ways, and the local and contingent practices of families that may, or may not, pull in other directions. This is not to suggest that either set of practices is in any sense 'pure' or clear and distinct – rather, the mix and mesh of discourse at work always also reflects relations to the social moment we are in, one that engages multiple collective frames including those of politics, economy and culture (Cohen, 1998). However, in this chapter our analytical task is to try to unweave the tangle of biomedical patterning and family arrangements, to follow family arrangements, and at the same time, to try to trace those elements from 'outside' their borders that become consequential in the continuing adjustment and maintenance of those arrangements (López, 2015). That is, to try, as López argues, to 'see' the mixings as they occur as well as the care needed to keep family arrangements 'functional and meaningful' (2015, p 92).

Family arrangements are essentially what support the practices and the people. All families have arrangements (and boundaries), even if they move. All arrangements have a certain composition, even if that changes and evolves, and all have relations with practices outside their borders that need to be continually qualified, requalified and changed (Thygesen and Moser, 2010). It is this last point in particular that is of concern for this chapter – living with a dementia implies profound changes in people and their relations with others, to family routines and other activities (Ceci et al, 2020). The suspicion and later diagnosis of a dementia brings with it certain 'things', things that were not 'there' before, and tensions may be generated in intersections and interferences (Moser, 2011) of divergent practices, shaping, reshaping and shifting family arrangements. The stories of this chapter show something of the work involved in keeping in sync with these shifts.

Aside from understanding better what may be at stake for families living with a dementia, why does this matter? In part, this matters because, as noted previously, the biomedical patterning of dementia is very powerful, and, in turn, patterns what is done, or thought should be done, when families turn to health and social care systems for assistance. Formal care systems are strongly patterned by a biomedical ethos and in some respects, getting help requires being aligned with this pattern, which, depending on family patterning, can be more or less consequential for families. As effects of organizing practices, biomedical patterning creates relations and divisions that work to institute variable possibilities for connection and disconnection (Spoelstra, 2005; Cooper and Law, 2016 [1995]; Parker, 2015). Some families may 'take on' these other practices, some may partially align their relations and priorities, while others may resist, and despite widely diverse thresholds for accommodating change in family members, probably all 'learn' what it is they need to pay attention to in seeking help from formal care systems. In this context, family patterns of doing dementia are, at the very least, a confounding variable for those formal practices that tend towards homogenizing experience in order to better plan and predict, but perhaps that element with most actual effect in terms of how care proceeds for people. Questions about these various patternings can be highlighted or left in the background, but if highlighted, they generate a complexity in understanding daily life in the context of dementia that can't be flattened out.

Helen and Albert and the 'beginnings of dementia'

This first story is about sense making and the work of patterning, and about the capacity of a biomedical patterning of ageing and dementia to draw in all sorts of people to think about and organize their lives in similar ways – people who are kind of 'like' the pattern, and kind of not like the pattern. Some of the patterning we see across the families involved in this research comes about because all were met in the same way – through Alzheimer's Society caregiver support groups. So these were families who self-identified as people dealing with something that was patterned in a particular way, including the patterning of 'caregiving' as something needing support and information. We start with Helen and Albert Baker, an older couple, together for many years and now struggling to understand Albert "behaving differently". Or at least this is something Helen and her children are trying to make sense of, as Albert does not see his various "troubles" as a problem.

Here we draw from an initial interview with Helen and Albert at the beginning of their involvement with the research. Helen and Albert got involved with this study because Helen believed that Albert had the "beginnings of dementia" and had support for this view from two of her daughters. What seems to be at stake here is Albert's decreasing ability to be organized. Helen says changes were first noticed about two years ago by their daughter, Alison, who worked at the family bookstore with Albert – she told her mum that sometimes Albert was misplacing orders, and while 'he always had a habit of putting stuff on little bits of paper', now these papers would disappear. The family dealt with this by having a family meeting to get Albert to stop working so much, and to let Alison take over the main part of the business. So Albert started going into the store less and less – which he says gave him less structure in his day, and made him feel even less organized. When Helen gives her version of these events, she acknowledges that Albert might not agree with her.

At the beginning, both Helen and Albert were a bit unclear as to whether Albert has been formally diagnosed with a dementia – she says yes; he says the doctor told him he "scored well"; she says he believes what he wants to believe, and so on. But Helen knows about "dementia" because her mother had dementia:

> 'Because my mom had dementia, but I was never really there, right, 'cause I lived here. So – and I've seen other people – well, and Albert's mom had dementia. So you know, they go from – and the doctor he explained it so nicely. He said, "Helen, there's three steps to it. Here is where they take medication and they go downhill, and they still go to the bottom here. And there's a third [of people] that say, 'Ah, it's okay', so they still go to the bottom." And he says, "Here's the one that don't want any [medication], and they go there, too. So in the end", he says, "all three [groups of people] will end up right there." So what are you going to do when somebody's stubborn, doesn't want medication, right? But nobody else has to explain it. I can see it myself. I know he has it, you know, 'cause I know things he doesn't do.' (Interview, September 2015)

In this excerpt, Helen is telling about a conversation with the family doctor, with whom she has shared concerns about Albert. She reports how the doctor has told her about "dementia", and how it progresses. From this conversation, and from her experience with other family members, she "knows" Albert has "it" – "it" would explain for her the changes she has seen. In any case, while it is not entirely clear yet what is going on, it seems fair to say that this is a family that has been experiencing some changes, changes that have concerned them to the extent that they have sought some kind of external explanation that might help. But the changes do seem vague, and it's hard for them to say exactly what has changed – especially when Albert is present. Sometimes they talk about him as being "in denial" – which is something that is almost impossible for him to refute. This underlines the acutely attributional nature of "dementia" with a diagnosis requiring both the presence of the "senile body", the body in which the disease is located, and "a second body that notices changes in the first" (Cohen, 1998, p 33). It is the second body that provides the essential legitimacy for diagnosis, contributing historical and situated knowledge of the person in time – Albert was like "this", but now he is like this. But in order for change to be interpreted and acted on as (possible) dementia, Cohen points us to a third body – the collective representation of dementia, a "fact" of/in the world, which relies, as Gubrium (1986) has also suggested, on the continual public enactment of dementia as a disease about which something should be done. Thus "changes" in Albert move outside the family and enter into dialogue with other worlds, including widely circulated information about the signs, stages and burdens of dementia that shape shared social understandings or stock knowledge (Schutz, 1946) about what to make of changes in memory and/or behaviour as one gets older. This dialogue with other worlds instigates, even propels, the family's action, including both seeking medical confirmation through testing and diagnosis and attendance at the Alzheimer's Society to help Helen prepare for what is coming. And so it is that the collective representation of dementia, one possible conceptual space available to make sense of Albert's changing behaviour, offers direction to this family as to how they should proceed.

What is "dementia" about for this couple, this family? How did Albert's "behaviour" – as this seems to be a concern – become a sign of dementia? And what is at stake for this family in understanding Albert as having a disease versus Albert growing older, somewhat slower and more forgetful? Both things seem to be going on here as Helen says one of the things she notices is that Albert does not like to be rushed because that confuses him, but then she adds, she doesn't like to be rushed either, she likes to do things in her own time. And Helen and Albert do share a stock of understandings about ageing, that is, both agree that forgetfulness is part of ageing (Albert says that "everybody loses a certain amount of memory with ageing, regardless" and Helen agrees "yeah I forget all the time"), but only Helen is drawing into their arrangements a widely available public discourse about the nature of dementia to describe the private troubles Albert is experiencing, troubles that could conceivably be understood as normal (Gubrium, 1986).

Part of what emerges in the initial interview is that both Helen and Albert have noticed changes in themselves – changes framed in terms of memory, cognition, the pace at which they carry out everyday activities. What is interesting is that Albert was perhaps never a highly organized man – he's always had his own system of little bits of paper – but with age and time his strategies are now seen as a sign of cognitive decline. While a possible road for Helen might have been to do nothing when she noticed changes in Albert, instead she is trying to improve something, to translate troubles that are loose and vague into something more stable, and importantly, about which something might be done (Gubrium and Järvinen, 2014). In some respects it seems that what Helen has been mainly facing is a problem of definition (Cooper, 2003), and in her reality-defining work she pulls in the materials of the world to translate her uncertainties into something if not entirely certain, at least somewhat more explicable. Dementia can be the 'thing' that makes Albert different – forgetful, losing things, less organized – a way to structure or make sense of the differences through an alternative, and hopefully effective, vocabulary, one that builds a bridge between their private troubles and improving these. Similar to the phenomena described by Gubrium (1986), the public discourse tells her something about how to feel about and act in relation to this disease. Albert's denials make no difference, becoming part of the signs of his disease. Yet Albert says he manages his forgetfulness – he puts his things in a certain place, and only if he is rushed does he forget where they are – thus it is not a problem for him. And, he asserts, if he doesn't change his clothes as often, something which Helen is reading as another sign of the disease, it's only because he is "not as fussy" as Helen.

It is this aspect of biomedical patterning of dementia, its transformational and performative effects, that we draw out of Helen and Albert's story. In connecting to a collective image and concern, these concerns are drawn down and interwoven with old, established patternings to make something new, and in so doing shift what is at stake in Helen and Albert's arrangements. This is, in many ways, a productive transformation, in the sense that it makes their world different; it produces new, albeit contested by some members, ways of relating, and implies new possibilities for intervening in daily life (Parker, 2015). To the extent that Helen has brought her concerns forward, she becomes an observer and assessor, continually on the look-out for "signs" of dementia in Albert because for Helen, "it's definitely there". She is now, or will soon be, a 'caregiver' for a person with dementia, and is already worried, anticipating a trajectory wherein, as she says, "things will get worse". For her there is now a caregiver support group, where she gleans information she assumes will help her to prepare for this new and riskier future. Identity shifting effects are also realized for Albert in his relations with this medicalized patterning (Star, 1990) – he is no longer, or not only, a somewhat forgetful, slightly disorganized man, but a 'person with dementia', someone who, despite his emphatic resistance, is anticipated by those around him to lose his ability to manage day-to-day life to the course of a disease. This knowledge and the practices that accompany it restructure daily life, and at the same time, invoke a moral world (Cohen, 1998) – 'changes' in Albert are now not something to live alongside but to actively take care of, reflecting a working belief that there is sense to be made, things to be done. And, in being transformed from people experiencing vague troubles to having a more certain problem, in first recognizing and then becoming aligned with the pattern, Helen and Albert are now set up for 'help'. As Gubrium and Järvinen (2014) suggest, in the world of formal care, help is always attached to a problem and not to the troubles of daily living.

Ken and Marla: 'your patient/my wife'

Making a connection to dementia discourse has world-changing effects for Helen and Albert's arrangements, beyond any changes Albert may be experiencing. They have 'signed on' (Star, 1990), albeit only partially, to well-established structures of formal care and support, a standardized and standardizing network of knowledge and practice that they may not fully need now, but that Helen has already learned to anticipate needing down the road. In recognizing the pattern, which as Cooper and Law (2016) suggest is also part of the patterning, they localize and stabilize some of the troubles they have been experiencing, working with and through a new frame of reference that promises to help them to anticipate, and possibly prepare for, a now at least partially 'known' future.

It was a different story for Ken and Marla Roberts. At the time they became involved in the research, 'dementia' was drawn deeply into their everyday lives, the realities of disease producing profound alterations in their relations and practices. Ken, when we first met, was pretty much at the end of his tether, struggling with the meaningfulness of his everyday life. He had worked it out like this: "we are awake for about 103 hours per week, I have 23 hours of respite, that means 80 hours a week of just me and her, and it's like living with a two-year-old" (Field notes, September 2015). Yet, while there were distressing changes in Marla, developing over many years, and probably equally, although differently distressing, changes in Ken, there was also the 'dementia trajectory'. Trajectory discourse appears in Ken and Marla's story as a central sense-making mechanism, having powerful organizing effects in their family arrangements. But also, and this is what is perhaps more interesting, it seemed to have other more strategic effects, used by Ken to mark out and manage the borders between family and formal care practices.

Ken had a practice of writing letters to Marla's doctor prior to appointments. There are eight of these letters, written between January 2012 and September 2015, giving an account of changes he observed in Marla and in their daily life, as well as describing unusual, sometimes distressing, events that had occurred. The letters are densely written, in most instances comprised of about two pages of single spaced text. The letters are also invariably addressed 'your patient/my wife', a hybrid turn of phrase expressing identities and experiences simultaneously separated and joined, one now being implicated in the articulation of the other. The framing also institutes action at a boundary that divides and connects at the same time (Spoelstra, 2005), what Cooper has written about as a 'labour of division', bound up with the act of seeing and founded in a logic of the 'between' (Cooper and Law, 2016; Cooper, 1997, 2003). The 'between' is neither one thing nor the other, but a space of action drawing together and mixing repertoires of different worlds (Star, 1990). The labour of division works in this space, separating things in order to arrange them, or, as Parker (2015, p 491) suggests, intervening to 'produce a world we can understand and work with'. In differentiating patient and wife, and at the same time relating these identities, surfaces touch but not completely, signalling new partial and precarious connections being made and unmade (Cooper and Law, 2016). In Ken's letters, a boundary relation is being formed – for example, between then and now, between clinic and home, between Marla as patient and Marla as wife – but it is mixed because these are not quite separable, the relations not quite clear. But Ken's form of attention starts to make a pattern – a Marla then and now that emerges from their relations, history and ways of doing daily life.

In the first letter Ken writes, '[The] following is a summary of my observations that have led me to believe that my wife Marla is beginning to suffer from some form of dementia' (January 2012). He contrasts how Marla used to be – active, engaged, social, able to sew her own clothes, plan and execute large dinner parties. But now 'she sits at home in her chair for most of the day with repetitive music playing in the background while thumbing through tabloid quality magazines or flyers which don't appear to influence her shopping decisions' (January 2012). The details of this letter are very specific, full of disparate examples of odd behaviour, or at least behaviour that differs from before. Another example: 'weekday meals are nearly always a repeat of the previous week and every day she suggests the same frozen yogurt for dessert with no interest in even making Jell-O, a pudding or even a simple cake' (January 2012). There is little obvious structure to this first letter; it is a running narrative, a story that offers a montage of events, behaviours and communicative difficulties that are clearly distressing and bewildering for Ken. He ends the letter, 'It's hard for me to know what to do! Do I ignore her allowing her to sink further into her trance-like state? Do I contradict her thereby reducing her self-confidence? How do I keep from getting angry with these repeated anomalies in our way of life?' (January 2012).

The concern Ken expresses in this letter is that things have changed – long-established and evidently cherished patterns of daily life are becoming disordered. For the outsider reading his words, the specificity of the details he includes marks their singularity – the things that are changing have relevance to his and Marla's way of life and to no one else. Marla reads flyers that don't influence her shopping decisions, she has little interest in desserts – behaviours that are not necessarily unusual in themselves, or textbook 'signs' of dementia, but in the Roberts' specific shared practices of daily life, they are signs of something going on – they are anomalies in their way of life. In the second letter, written in May 2013, it seems clear that Ken has been given or found a way to make some sense of these anomalies. This letter, also written in preparation for an upcoming doctor's appointment, is differently organized. This letter has headings: 'My observations', 'Communications', 'Areas of concern'. His observations are now in point form and expressed in more 'objective', even clinical, terms: 'Obsesses over simple tasks and unable to organize or prioritize a series of them, then frantically jumps from one to another' (May 2013). There are still hints of the specificities of their daily life, for example, 'When grocery shopping she periodically strays from the list that I prepare, variously buying double or half the normal quantity that we need or on a whim picking something up that we may never get around to using' (May 2013). But by the third letter in November 2013, these hints of daily life become more muted, with Ken's earlier concern with 'anomalies' in their shared way of living replaced by new headings and new concerns: 'Potential malnutrition?' 'Personal hygiene?' 'Bathroom habits?' (November 2013).

In April 2014 Ken writes a letter outlining his goal for an upcoming doctor's appointment: 'The main purpose of this visit is to explore my concern that Marla has advanced to Middle Stage Alzheimer's in the last year as many of the concerns I've previously made you aware of have become much more prevalent' (April 2014). This letter also includes a copy of an information pamphlet from the local Alzheimer's Society that describes the effect of dementia on language ability. Ken has highlighted text in two colours – signs evident to him shortly after Marla's initial diagnosis and updated with a different colour representing changes in the two years since then (February 2014).

The final four letters are written between October 2014 and September 2015. In October he writes, 'My concerns that Marla is well into Middle Stage Alzheimer's are growing as she continues to devolve.' His January 2015 letter includes a note of recent MMSE scores, and increasingly technical language – he is now concerned that she has an 'Auditory Processing Disorder: Marla rarely understands anything I say to her and consequently doesn't respond.' He then writes, 'I'm concerned that Marla is into "late middle stage" and am concerned about how I will I know when it's time for her to live in a care facility.' In May 2015 he writes, 'Due to my observations over the last three months, I have deep concerns that Marla has slipped from Middle Stage into Late Stage Alzheimer's and that she soon won't be able to continue living at home with me' (May 2015). This letter, as with all the others, includes detailed descriptions of his work of attending to Marla's personal hygiene, including dealing with periodic incontinence, as well as his challenges in keeping their home tidy or preparing Marla for outings. He is much preoccupied with the impossibilities of maintaining even the simplest of their usual routines and practices – with these troubles offered as further evidence of decline.

In most of the later letters, Marla appears mostly as 'patient', described in terms of shifting capacities and the troubles these present for Ken. In the representation of his observations, he draws in and implicates the doctor as an expert on these concerns, in a sense using the trajectory patterning to establish lines of responsibility: 'The list goes on and on but I'll stop here and hope that these notes give you areas to explore for her future wellbeing.' He ends this letter, as well as the final letter written in September, with evident despair: 'I've had to abandon many of my own activities so we spend days locked in our home with nothing to do or even talk about on days when she's not at her day programme'.

Our interest in sharing Ken's letters is not that they tell the whole story, but that as a technology of representation, the letters, by their very nature, have required action from Ken in terms of an imposition of order, a patterning of experience. That is to say, there are many styles of writing, many forms of attention, many possibilities for inclusion and exclusion in the telling of stories. Ken's actions of selection, attention and emphasis in his letters can be seen as one way he is trying to make sense, to stabilize, to institute at least the appearance of control over an experience that is much larger than he is able to represent. So in this labour of division, choices must be made as to what to represent, where his efforts should be directed. That he is writing these letters to the doctor is significant, as after the first letter, he organizes his experience in a way that it may hopefully be better read and understood.

However even Ken's first letter, which is looser, more narrative in form, shows effort to fix action and behaviour – this was Marla 'then'; this is Marla 'now'. A process of division is happening that begins the making of a new object, a hybrid – 'your patient/my wife'. Although he has not yet fixed on a clear framework within which to situate his troubles – the 'anomalies' disrupting his and Marla's shared way of living – the letter begins the work of division necessary to discerning pattern. But as Chia (1998) notes, in the action of representing, writing is also a social process of world making, helping to generate the patterned regularities that are then amenable to re-presentation. This labour of division has consequences, producing an orderly story of (apparent) disorder and working to direct Ken's attention in specific ways. Or, as Foucault (2003, p xv) suggests, it is to employ an anterior gaze that seems to 'turn darkness into light'; once the trajectory framework is in place, progression through stages is observable. To notice the influence of biomedical patterning in Ken's letters is not to suggest this is good or bad, but to consider what it leads to, how it is helpful and/or what it helps with.

One of the ways Ken's attention shifts through the letters is in the pairing of 'your patient/my wife'. The first letter seems clearly to do with Marla, his wife, and how things are changing for them. This shifts as the letters become more aligned with organized representations of Marla's decline, serving to fix her in relation to a biomedical patterning of dementia – stages are fitted to behaviours and behaviours are fitted to stages, and all changes are localized within Marla. A trajectory of regular monitoring measures change, but also frames the changes that will be noticed and reported. Although Ken continues to address the letters 'your patient/my wife', the former term seems to govern the latter as Ken begins to include mainly those details relevant to the biomedical pattern – communicative difficulties, cognitive symptoms, specific activities of daily living (ADLs), responses to medications. Observing these details rather than others, and rendering them in biomedical phrasing helps them to 'travel' to become part of Marla's regular medical appointments, and as quoted previously, performs another labour of division, signalling to the doctor both what Ken's responsibilities are but also what belongs to the medical world. He gives the doctor that 'material' which should help the doctor to help Marla and himself to respond 'medically' to the evidently 'medical' details of their experience.

In order to be taken seriously, and also perhaps to guide the doctor's attention, Ken has somewhere learned that he needs to assemble these details into a pattern recognizable within a biomedical framing – at some point he has been 'persuaded' to order his observations in this way. As Cooper and Law (2016, p 216) argue, such patterning is 'recursively intentional'. That is, biomedical patterning of dementia, by transforming messy and disordered experience into discrete and explicable problems, works to order experience along those same line – it works anteriorly (Foucault, 2003) to show Ken how to give an account of his and Marla's lives that can be taken seriously by those who are presumably in a position to help. Biomedical patterning performs knowledge – this, then this, then this – stages marked by declining numbers, and a sense of movement towards a destination of some sort. Attaching Marla's decline to a known trajectory seems to help Ken; it offers a way to organize his present and his future, a path and a sense of timing (Gubrium, 1986). The trajectory also lets Ken know that, at a certain point, he will have 'permission' to detach as caregiver, an 'inevitable' outcome of the timing and staging of the disease. As Ken notes in his May 2015 letter, it is Marla's now evidencing signs of 'late stage Alzheimer's' that will explain her transition to an institutional care setting.

While Ken seems to use his letters to direct the actual 'clinical gaze' of the doctor, drawing boundaries between his own care practices and where help is needed, it is also worth noting that an effect of the gaze Ken employs to accomplish this also positions him as an external, deciphering subject (Foucault, 2003), with Marla the object of his attentions. The careful cataloguing of her behaviour, signs and symptoms performs Marla as an instance of more general knowledge, attending mainly to the ways she is 'like' the pattern. As Marla is produced as a 'case', Ken is relegated to itemizing and tracking her decline, her movement along this trajectory. In the end, however, or perhaps simply in life, Marla is not a case, and the careful labour of division seems to collapse as the situation reasserts itself: 'I've abandoned all my own activities so we spend days locked in our home, sometimes with her in her nightie and housecoat all day with nothing to do or even talk about on days when she's not at her day programme or home care workers are not present' (September, 2015). The biomedical patterning, carefully drawn in and made use of for so long to order the experience, is no longer so useful. The patterning may help to 'locate' or 'package' the person, but in the end there is care for and life with this person – and the pattern does not help much with this. Rather, we hear Ken's plea: we are trapped here together, *this* is what is at stake for us – not so much 'knowing' what is going on, but thinking what can be done.

What can be done turns out to be somewhat limited. During the next clinic appointment Marla's doctor has read Ken's last letter and expresses concern about how Ken is managing:

FIELD NOTES
September 2015

Ken says 'the main thing is for me to get time to myself.' The doctor asks, 'Is it something you'd be willing to pay for?' Ken replies 'The bigger issue is that we're awake for 100 hours a week, I have 23 hours of respite, that leaves us with 80 hours, two shifts a day all week.' The doctor says, 'We can't get away from that – we talked last time about Memantine [medication used to treat moderate to severe Alzheimer's disease] – it helps with compliance – studies show it can release your time trying to get things done by about an hour a day– it costs about $150/month – that's about $5/day.' Ken says 'The problem is, I'm trapped'. The doctor suggests the drug might decrease some of Ken's frustration and asks whether some of the tasks could be put to home care. Ken says 'Respite is what I'm really after – I need a week.' The doctor says 'We can put that in our letter to home care – to triage you highly, and that you need respite for a week at a time.' Ken tells her that the case manager has already told him there is no week-long respite available in the near term – 'Maybe next year, she said'.

Later that same day Ken receives a call at home from the transition coordinator telling him that Marla can be "fast tracked" for placement. In describing this conversation he says it is "shocking how fast this has happened", but he is also almost jubilant; "finally", he says, "we are all on the same page now" (Field notes, September 2015).

In reading over Ken's letters, it seems clear that part of Ken's handling of dementia has been to track Marla's "progress" along a trajectory, first "learning" the trajectory, including its relation to formal care system supports, and in this way learning the future. On the one hand, we see the extent of the work, struggles and tensions entailed in living with a person with a dementia. On the other, we can see how the "work" itself has been shaped in important ways by how the healthcare system is organized. Support has been linked to stages: first, there is information and education and medication to forestall symptoms, then the day programme, then in-home assistance and a few hours of respite, then an offer of more medication to control symptoms, longer periods of respite (*if* it is available) – and through all of this is the foregrounded concern to keep Marla and then Ken "going" for as long as possible. This suite of supports is not unusual, comprised of episodic interventions to elongate time in the community and to delay institutionalization. In the moment, and from the "outside", this arrangement seems to play out in hard ways for families like Ken and Marla, leaving Ken to "work", as he says, two shifts a day for seven days a week (Field notes, September 2015). But it also seems to have become normalized, expected and accepted. As Ken says much later, several months after Marla is moved out of their home, he thinks they have had a "pretty acceptable journey compared to some".

FIELD NOTES
November 2015
He goes on to say, 'There is no technical reason she [Marla] couldn't still live at home – she was safe, still eating, I was toileting her and taking care, with home care, of the personal hygiene.' I ask if this was about needing to look after himself, but he doesn't answer.

In some respects this takes us back to López (2015, p 92) and the care needed to keep family arrangements both 'functional and meaningful'. At stake seem to be practices that, as families 'move' along the dementia trajectory, ensure their eventual reordering as sets of 'caregivers' and 'care recipients', with home unmade and then remade to function as a space of healthcare rather than a place of everyday life. Ken's words quoted earlier reveal the extent to which their home had become repatterned as an institutional world, and the relations therein reshaped as 'technical'. But at the same time this has not been accomplished without suffering, the 'ecology of home' profoundly altered as it is permeated by the logic of formal care practices (Star, 1990, p 379), including, as care crumbled, the identities of both Ken and Marla.

Ken and Marla's "acceptable journey" led them to a place of seeming "mere" functional existence. It was a highly medicalized trajectory, moved in part by Marla's particular experience of dementia, but also how the conceptual space of a medicalized trajectory worked with this couple. As well as laying out the presumed course of disease, the trajectory discourse signalled and enacted a policy of delaying institutionalization, with everyone involved doing their part to accomplish this goal. In Ken's case there were things this discourse helped with. It offered him a formal language to share his experience with those he saw as positioned to help him, it enabled a structuring of system resources and expectations, and it pointed to an 'end' helping to mediate the psychological wrenching of Marla from Ken and their home. The trajectory discourse also did work in bridging a division – 'your patient/my wife' – enabling the new and alienating requirement to live in multiple worlds (Star, 1990). But we do tend to lose track of Marla in this story except as a problem to be solved – as much work as the pattern does to impose some order on life, it must also be the case that a lot of life escapes or evades the pattern.

Colleen and James and being prepared

To the extent that a family's everyday practices are already deeply patterned (Schutz, 1944; Straßheim, 2016), a family member 'behaving differently' to an intolerable degree requires not only explanation but also new patterning to accommodate change. Dementia trajectory patterning is, in a sense, 'ready to use', providing both the needed explanation and a new plan. It tells people fairly explicitly how to perform the role of 'caregiver' for a certain sort of person, laying out what they are being asked to do and for (approximately) how long. But, as noted previously, there are various possibilities for connection and disconnection to the dementia trajectory, having to do with previously established patterns, histories and ways of doing daily life. There is also the varied tolerance for 'behaving differently', in some part related to just what that behaviour entails, but also to a family's varied strategies and capacities for accommodation.

The possibility of aggressive behaviour is probably one of the most difficult to accommodate (Ceci et al, 2018b). When Colleen and James Miller became involved in the study, they had already been living with James' diagnosis of a dementia for about two years, and a central concern shaping daily life was what Colleen described as James' "volatility". What could be done was somewhat limited. There were changes to be made in routines, staying alert to what overwhelmed James, looking out for the possibility he might become frustrated or tired and lash out. There were practices of "redirecting", distracting James, turning his attention or focus away from whatever had agitated him. There was the day programme placement extended to three days a week to give Colleen and James at least some time apart and decrease the "friction" between them. There was also medication to "tamp down" his temper, but the trade-off was he might become more "muddled", which might also make him feel overwhelmed and angry. But these strategies were somewhat uncertain – dependent on

Colleen's abilities to read James and the situations they are in. And so many variables – the time of day, what activities they are doing, and where they are – everything in play all the time.

For Colleen, trajectory discourse provided a kind of ready-made blueprint to manage these uncertainties. Since James' diagnosis she had actively sought information – taking several courses about dementia, including a correspondence course on "dealing with dementia" and how to be a caregiver. She says, "I am always looking for a course that can help" (Field notes, March 2015). She attended several different caregiver support groups, although in the end she found these less useful, saying she was frustrated with people's lack of "urgency". She says she tells other caregivers to make a plan: "do it sooner because later your plate is going to be full" (Field notes, September 2015). She had also collected a vast amount of information – two 4-inch binders filled with pamphlets from many sources on topics such as how to best handle dementia 'behaviours', how to access community resources, as well as managing financial and legal concerns. A reason she gives for this collection is that she is always asking herself "am I missing something?" (Field notes, March 2015). She also keeps a notebook with a record of all her contacts with the formal health system, including James' doctor and case manager. In all of this work, Colleen had resourcefully gathered together what she assumed to be the "known" elements of the trajectory, working from a "playbook" about how this disorder should be perceived and acted on. A key here, as with the previous stories, is the notion of anteriority – knowing in advance what to expect would help Colleen to "be prepared".

If the 'dementia trajectory' tells a story about how a person will change, it also provides a 'template' that tells of how to be a 'successful caregiver'. The courses, the support groups, the binders of information all suggest there is an expertise or mastery to be achieved, a more or less well-defined programme of knowledge for 'dementia caregiving' that is separate from the knowledge a person uses in other family roles. As well as positioning Colleen and James and their relationship in a new way, Colleen's knowledge of the 'dementia trajectory' performs a structure that is helpful to her – the notebooks, binders, and courses allow her to make something that runs (mostly) smoothly.

Colleen is a good manager; she is organized, and prepared, she has done her homework. She has worked hard, in the face of James' uncertain and sometimes scary behaviours, to shape their world in at least somewhat predictable ways. It is hard not to be struck with the overwhelming organizing effects of Colleen's work, with so many different pieces needing to be working together to keep this all in line – family care practices must work with formal care practices, day programmes must be available to 'hold' James at least some of the time, doctors must be available to offer medication advice and help Colleen know how to manage risks, and institutional placement must be available when these risks become untenable. For Colleen, some of her ability to 'care' relies on the extent to which she can align her work with a system that she interacts with as her 'partner' in care. A doctor's appointment offers an opportunity to show this alignment, and also for Colleen to become visible as a resourceful person:

FIELD NOTES

March 2015

Colleen brings out her notebook and begins recounting a number of incidents since the last appointment. The concern for the doctor and for Colleen is that James is 'becoming a little more challenging'. Colleen says he can be 'explosive', which has now been witnessed by other family members. The doctor says, placement is the 'looming issue' and they talk together about possibilities, with Colleen telling the doctor that she has already been working to arrange tours of facilities.

There is more conversation where Colleen describes more incidents and she and the doctor try to "problem-solve" James' "breaking point". They also discuss the effects of a medication they are trying to manage James' "temper" – it's hard to tell, says Colleen, if the medication has helped – so many factors are involved. After a while the doctor says:

FIELD NOTES

March 2015

'You are doing an incredible job' – then she turns to a student doctor also in the room to say, 'She has done so much to educate herself.' Colleen says 'Ignorance is not bliss' and that knowledge gives her a capacity to deal with things. After a pause the doctor says, 'He is not the James you married'. Colleen nods.

Perhaps we can see here why Colleen has done so much work to "educate" herself – at times James can be difficult to predict, a threat to her safety. Is it this that has "flipped" her into the caregiver role so firmly, a situation that requires such careful management? Her work here is praised by the doctor – she is a model caregiver, educating herself, working to prevent problems, being proactive. At the same time there are ways that we can see that James has been constituted as an "object of work" for Colleen – that a record is kept of him, and his activities are reported on and discussed in terms of signs and symptoms, possible interventions. This is a clinical repertoire. Yet at the same time, part of the work being done here is to improve Colleen's life, to support her and keep her going – so, although enacting caregiver, she is, simultaneously, an object of concern.

In some ways, the interaction here echoes Ken Roberts' comment from the previous story – everybody seems to be on the same page, although it must be noted that being on the same page seems to need James to start to be detached in some way from Colleen. And, like Ken, Colleen appears to have "learned" what she needs to pay attention to, to get help from the system. More so than Ken, however, Colleen seems to have taken on the concerns of the healthcare system and made them her own. She has done a tremendous amount of organizing work on behalf of the system, been independent, not asked for too much help and in many ways, managed their own trajectory even to the point of starting to investigate possible institutional placements on her own.

But even with all this effective organization, there is precarity in Colleen and James' arrangements. This becomes apparent a few weeks later when the 'system', in effect, lets her down. Colleen tells the following story:

FIELD NOTES
April 2015

The coordinator of James' day programme called to report that James had started screaming at another patient while waiting for the bus to come home. This was another man who 'agitates' James – they are usually kept apart but somehow that hadn't happened on this day. Questions were raised as to whether James would be able to continue going to the day programme. The coordinator called again the next Friday, and said that Colleen should have James 'checked out' by the family doctor. A plan was made for Colleen to accompany James to the day programme as an 'observer'. But before that could happen there was another incident over lunch at the programme and James became agitated. The staff of the day programme talked and they made the decision to discharge James from the day programme, and then called Colleen to inform her of this. Colleen called her case manager, her family doctor and the geriatrician. She couldn't reach her case manager, the doctors don't work Fridays. Says the situation was difficult for her because it was 'a decision I didn't make' –'they just called and informed me what they were going to do.'

Colleen says "a crisis hit" and she expected "people to respond" – but instead, she is faced with people she had carefully cultivated over the past number of months who are not responding properly to her situation, people who have made decisions without her input and, who, as a result, have decreased her options. She has invested so much time and effort into being prepared, and now all these people are letting her down, just when she most needs them. She goes on to say, "I was very upset that they discharged him, that choices were taken away from me." Then she says, "I realized I was treating this like a job; this is my job, but I am not in control of it" (Field notes, April 2015). At some point, to "go on" in this situation, Colleen had created a careful structure – a space in which she can manage either James' behaviour or his possible behaviour. She has sought and valued control, but it is a problem that this structure is somewhat brittle – events happen and all will depend on relations with other people and systems that are not, perhaps, working in the same way she is. She has kept faith with the trajectory discourse, a patterning of relations, time and events that promised her knowledge and perhaps a means of securing the future, but it does not quite deliver.

Interferences and intersections

What can we learn from our attempts to 'unweave' 'dementia trajectory' discourse and the kinds of practices this implies, from daily life with a dementia? As one would expect, the families whose stories we've told here were all very different, dealing with singular constellations of troubles and concerns, even if these get put under the same general name – they had their own patterning, their own practices, were different in terms of thresholds of what could and could not be accommodated, and different in terms of how a biomedical patterning of dementia was to be related to and worked with. In each case, however, relations needed to be made. With Helen and Albert we see the narrowness of the conceptual space afforded them in making sense of changes as they aged. Although Albert resists, a biomedical patterning of this experience is difficult to withstand, and trajectory discourse changes what is at stake in their relations, mobilizing a new and different repertoire of living with uncertainty. For Ken and Marla, the pattern becomes a hinge between home and clinic, and a way to insistently direct the expert clinical gaze to their troubles, to show what needed to be taken care of "medically". But at the same time, it also shifts and clinicalizes Ken's gaze, makes Marla a "case" to be known in a particular way, but that doesn't really help much in the end when there is care for this person, and someone has to do it and it is experienced as an endless task. But then the task is not endless, even when the end does seem to come about somewhat arbitrarily. And for Colleen, the standardized patterning told her how to "be prepared", how to planfully interact with and even structure system resources, how to be resourceful and "successful" in what she eventually realized had become a "job" – but not really. The efficiency and effectiveness of her work made her a "model" caregiver, and at the same time, in part because of the ways alliances were made to shift, shaped quite separate worlds for her and James.

Of course, this summing up misses a lot. And this, we think, is probably the most important observation – there is so much going on in the daily lives of families that even when trajectory discourse is working hard, there is still so much life that escapes the pattern – or perhaps more to the point, there is a big excess of life being pushed out by a focus on patterning. While this is not a surprising observation, we do think it is one worth hesitating over (Stengers, 2005b). From Mol et al (2010) we learn that any practice brings about both *goods* and *bads*, and that they have to be dealt with together. In family practices of living with a dementia there is being with, coming apart, caring for and being exhausted. There are old and new attachments, as well as things that become detached and lost. There is being "prepared", but then surprises, events happen. And in this mix there is 'the dementia trajectory', a somewhat narrow but increasingly common method to articulate and enact understandings of the situations families are dealing with. To the extent that trajectory discourses tend to make what Law and Urry (2004) would describe as a 'flat' or one-dimensional world, and do so in an overwhelming way, these ways of thinking 'dementia' have the potential (and power) to unmake and remake in helpful and not so helpful ways a family's historical and singular arrangements for living day to day. To be clear, the problem we see here is not so much the need a family may have to make new relations in light of a diagnosis of a dementia, but rather, the possibility of a 'life'-limiting sameness lived out in a too heavy reliance on the 'single story' that emerges from trajectory discourse.

At the same time, there were things that the trajectory discourse seemed to help with, mostly stemming from its anteriority. It pointed to an 'end', a course of events that would lead there, and a suite of formal care supports that would be available along the way. It showed how the practice of 'delaying institutionalization' could unfold, and provided 'reasons' for institutionalization that could, perhaps, be lived with. But even if this anteriority constitutes a 'good' for families, there also seems to be a point at which biomedical patterning stops working. For instance, at the point of 'caregiving', that space of looking at what needs to be done and how – that's where trouble starts to arise, trouble that comes, in part, because the 'plan' is based on something other than the singular life. The pattern seems to offer some sense of certainty, but in the family stories told here, uncertainty persists, in part because in its instantiation the standard pattern still relies on the images and concerns of a different world (Star, 1990). This raises a question – are trajectory discourses good ways to think what is going on for families?

On the one hand, framing people through an at least partly known progression of a disease may make it easier for formal care systems to help them; it can help to make families at least 'operationally visible' to the practices of professionals (Cooper, 1997, p 38). But, as Cooper also argues, drawing on Foucault's (1977) work on discipline, this enhanced visibility, 'a phenomenon of organized perception', is a disciplining gaze. Families may become more visible to professionals, and to the system itself, but mainly as 'cases' (Cooper, 1997, p 37). So there is a cost to be borne here as well. That is to say, in sighting families as 'cases' of something more general, the capacity to understand and respond to the singularity of family arrangements is much diminished. And if the work that families are doing is taking care of their arrangements, relating to rather than progressing along or managing a trajectory, have the possibilities for helping with this been prematurely shut down?

7

Borders and helpfulness

This chapter explores borders, and the relations of helping that happen both inside and outside of these borders, and perhaps most important, about the 'logic of the between' (Cooper and Law, 2016, p 207) that works to constitute various and precarious thresholds between these locations. We start with an idea, in many respects rather obvious, that we cannot use a term like 'help' with preconceived notions about what help means – that it is not really known in advance what 'help' will look like for a particular family. As Büscher and his colleagues (2011) have shown, in the context of evidence that current formal care practices and policies often create rather than resolve problems for families, helpfulness must be rethought in terms of how particular 'helping' actions fit, or don't fit, with ongoing family arrangements (Büscher et al, 2011, p 713; see also Lloyd and Stirling, 2011; Stirling et al, 2014; O'Shea et al, 2017; Stephan et al, 2018). Care for family arrangements draws us immediately to consideration of what is 'between' these and 'other' practices, and that is always something to find out about. In this chapter we develop this idea by drawing on Cooper and Law's distinction between proximal and distal analyses to explore the question of helpfulness through looking at details – materials, knowledges, technologies, policies and people, and importantly, the relations made among all of these – to understand 'help' as an effect of complex processes that 'take up, form and reform all these bits and pieces' (Cooper and Law, 2016, p 214). To show this idea, we describe processes and events that, in three of the participant families, sometimes led to 'help' as an effect, and sometimes did not.

We tie our analysis in this chapter to the idea of profound changes happening over time for families, changes often ending with family members relinquishing responsibility for daily care for the person living with dementia to paid staff in a residential care facility, even while still working out new ways of maintaining a relevant relationship in the spaces available in that new home. This change in living arrangements is profound, it happens in time, it happens differently in different families, and it is a process that draws and informs the attention of many of the 'helpful' actions of formal care systems. As we have shown in the previous two chapters, the change in living arrangements does not happen according to a simple and rational time frame despite its apparent alignment with a manufactured trajectory of disease progression. Instead, the transformation of a person who previously contributed to the definition of the family's trajectory in the world becomes someone whose day-to-day safety must be monitored and whose performance in contributing to daily activities such as meal preparation or personal care is measured against a 'dementia trajectory' that claims to inform families and professional care staff about pathways out of the family home and into a residential care placement. In this chapter we show three families' practices of living at home and in their community, how these practices come to be supported in particular ways by people and programmes representing professional support that is meant to help sustain the family in their home, and then how decisions to transfer the person diagnosed with dementia to a residential care facility are accomplished – a point that could be said to represent the 'limits' of helpfulness. However, to identify a limit condition is not to suggest that this is a fixed moment in time, a clearly recognizable endpoint – although there is much research interest in identifying the specific constellation of factors that could predict this event (Afram et al, 2015; Kelaiditi et al, 2016). Rather, the limit itself seems to be something that moves through and with practices and processes of helping until help, whatever that may be, no longer helps to sustain a particular family. In order to render some transparency to this process we focus on ideas that have been presented in earlier chapters, and here show how diverse practices operate to accomplish this significant event of a family member no longer belonging at home.

First, we introduce a new concept – that of the 'borders of helpfulness'. With this phrase we point towards relationships of exchange operating at the figurative threshold of the home, where family members who contribute to maintaining the home as a place where the person living with dementia lives, interact with formal care supports, including people and programmes arrayed throughout the community, occasionally crossing the threshold of the home with offers of help for family members doing the daily work of caring. Our interest in 'borders' initially arose from Stengers pressing the significance of thinking 'practices *among* practices', and the necessity this idea entails of considering how divergent practices might relate (Savransky and Stengers, 2018; see also Chapter 5). At the same time, we don't take the idea of borders as unproblematic, as pointing to 'invisible walls' dividing family and formal care practices (Cooper and Law, 2016, p 199). As Cooper and Law argue, to assume fixed states of being would be to attribute an 'already there', finished character to borders. Instead, we use the idea of borders to point to thresholds where there may be an 'inside' and 'outside' that holds the requirement of making relations, often enacted through the 'bits and pieces' noted earlier, and which directs us to consider what Cooper and Law describe as the 'logic of the between' (2016, p 207). This, they suggest, is 'where the action is' – a space that simultaneously 'divides and joins' so that connections are always, and can only be, 'partial and precarious' (2016, p 207). They cite historian of science James Gleick (1988, p 207) on this point: 'surfaces in contact do not touch everywhere'. The 'borders of helpfulness' then emerge as an effect of uncertain processes, that may or may not touch where needed, but are constituted proximally through various and ongoing possibilities for contact and motion. 'Border' functions here, as suggested by Cooper and Law, as an 'intervening medium, point or line of passage for action' (2016, p 201), or in our analysis here, a line of passage for 'help'. Central is consideration of the nature of the relations working at surfaces, when precarious connections may be held together to constitute 'help' as 'help', as well as instances when something perceivable as 'helpful' does not seem to occur. At that point of precarious connection, help offered, accepted, incorporated, accommodated, adjusted or rejected makes an inside and an outside conceivable, it marks a border (Starobinski, 1975). In his essay examining the hermeneutic task of understanding texts, Starobinski writes about the importance of thinking carefully about borders, about insides and outsides. He argues that when reading ancient texts, he prefers to 'preserve their foreignness, their exteriority intact' (p 336) so as not to take for granted a coherent tracing of meaning from historical use into present reading. He argues that '[n]o inside is conceivable, therefore, without the complicity of an outside on which it relies … [n]o outside would be conceivable without an inside fending it off, resisting it, "reacting" to it' (p 342). It is this location at the border between inside and outside, this 'place of exchanges, of adjustments' but also 'the place of conflicts or wounds' (p 342) that we also seek to preserve – in order to describe – as the borders of helpfulness. Just as Starobinski seeks to preserve the 'foreignness' of the ancient text, we analyse the accounts of families seeking help in a similar fashion: preserving as foreign both what families seek out as help as well as that offered to them as help by animate and inanimate objects.

Our argument as we lay it out in this chapter is that the operation of these relations of exchange across the threshold of the home plays a key part in both constituting that border of helpfulness between families and professional care providers as well as mobilizing the transformation of the person living with dementia in their home, ultimately accomplishing the movement of that person into a residential care situation. The removal of a family member from the family home is often a highly charged situation for everyone involved in the circumstance – one that can result in 'conflicts or wounds'. And yet, for the families involved in this study, the move seemed to occur relatively smoothly and without much of the overt conflict that such a significant intervention might be expected to cause. It is our view that the smoothing out of these activities as an event in the family's history occurs in good part as a result of years of groundwork accomplished at borders by both family members and formal care providers.

For instance, in Chapter 5 we showed how a focus on the notion of safety directed families to learn how best to accommodate the progressive changes they encountered in living with their family member diagnosed with dementia. These changes contribute to the smoothing out of the pathway leading towards institutionalization. As a point of contact between surfaces, discourses of safety raise questions in the minds of family members about whether the person living with dementia can be left alone at home anymore. It means that family members adjust their schedules so that one member of the family is always home to monitor the activities of the person living with dementia, to help them up when they fall and, over time, to not only watch their activities from afar, but to move in more closely to prevent the person from falling in the first place. So safety is one of the ideas that is exchanged across borders that works as part of a trajectory discourse shaping helping practices at home and, in so doing, articulates the specific vocabulary of the relations of exchange that will underpin some forms of help between formal care services and family members. As noted in Chapter 5, the idea that 'safety is most important' creates patterns of actions from both families and formal care providers that may simultaneously be in tension and work to hold these distinct practices together.

In Chapter 6 we showed how, when interfacing with formal care providers, families participated in watching for, describing and monitoring patterns of behaviour that helped to make some of their daily concerns visible to healthcare providers. For instance, through his careful documentation of Marla's daily activities, Ken described changes in Marla from someone active, engaged and very social, to someone who had become increasingly disengaged from the previous routines of their daily life together. Ken's monitoring of Marla's 'dementia trajectory' shows him taking on a new way of seeing Marla, one more characteristic of a biomedical or clinical gaze, looking for patterns and systematizing his observations in order to know better what was going on, and if possible, to find someone who could intervene or help (Foucault, 2003). Although each family related to the biomedical patterning of dementia in different ways, in each instance these relations made the families themselves more visible to formal care providers as 'cases' on which planning for a pathway towards a residential care can occur. Here, again, we can bring forward into this chapter the ideas of patterning and their contributory efforts to the development of a dementia trajectory to examine how tracking this trajectory is helpful to families and how it is also – and perhaps differently – helpful to formal care providers.

Safety concerns, events that help families see and then monitor patterns of behaviour framed as signs of progressively deteriorating cognitive ability – these are influential discursive practices that are mobilized to create access to homes where everyday care for people living with dementia occurs. If a family can be convinced that their family member with dementia is in danger, then security measures such as walking frames, commodes, and surveillance practices can be suggested and implemented in the home. When the person living with dementia is shown as someone no longer able to dress appropriately or be willing to take a shower, these actions can be reframed as signs of deterioration. Located somewhere along a trajectory of progressive illness, the person can be seen more easily as a person in need of help – and, through negotiating the logic of the between, paid caregivers might now be introduced, people who will come to the home two or three times a week, and who will, over time, start making daily visits to assist the person with a shower and to get dressed. Commodes, care aides, walking frames – these can be thought of as the materials of helping that the formal care system brings to the threshold of the home. These materials of helping do not work on their own; they must be brought into the home and put into practice by family members, by the person living with dementia and, at times, by formal care providers themselves when invited into the home. Those materials and practices, once inside the home, may operate as intended or may be used in quite unique ways, depending on the interests of the family.

And here is another idea presented earlier that we bring in again to this chapter, that of interests. The interests that families enact in helping their family member who lives with dementia are complex, multiple and diverse. In the sections that follow, we examine instances of those interests as they were enacted through language and actions during the time we spent with the families. This is an understanding of interests that draws on Cooper and Law's (2016, p 208) discussion of intention, where intention refers not to purely 'mental events' but to things that are 'in tension' responding to the pull and play of action. Similarly, in our analysis of the 'interests' of families, we are not only referring to desires or wants, but rather the ways these reference, reflect and constitute 'patterns of actions distributed throughout a field and which serve to maintain it or hold it together' (Cooper and Law, 2016, p 208). How a practice is 'held together' represents how the distinctive interests of a family are working, and shows something of that to which they are attached and that which attaches them to their specific practices. Formal care providers have interests too – in the families as well as specific interests in the person diagnosed with dementia, an interest that provides organizational legitimacy for their occasional presence in the home and their ongoing relationship with the family. These interests are also multiple, and maintain and hold together their own fields of action. So people living with dementia, those who care for them in their homes and formal care providers who suggest practices that might help or offer materials intended to support care processes – are all bespoke by interests. As we have suggested in previous chapters, in Stengers' (2019, p 60) ecological framing, although families and formal care providers may be thought as 'related by common interests', their distinctive practices work against common interests being the 'same' interests, even when it is the case that these 'diverging interests now need each other'.

And this is the core of our argument. In our descriptions of the borders of helpfulness instituted by family members and formal care providers as they engage in practices of exchange through which 'help' is sometimes actualized, an interest in the dementia trajectory creates a relation of 'common interest' between families and formal care provision – but this common interest does not mean they have the same interests in common. It does mean that diverging interests may now need each other. It is important to note, however, that in thinking with Stengers (2019, p 188), even in the context of such 'connecting events', our situation remains one of relational heterogeneity wherein those implicated in partial relations or 'connections in the making' 'go on diverging, go on in defining in their own manner what matters for them'. Thus the 'interests' involved are neither neutral nor general, and the rapport, or alignment, that sometimes develops is not innocent. Interests, suggests Stengers, are political and pragmatic, a question of 'who is, or will be affected, and how?' (2019, p 190). Asking this question is important as it gives to the situation the power to matter in a particular rather than a general way, it addresses people as they belong to a particular practice, which means addressing them in terms of their particular interests and attachments (Stengers, 2019, p 190). And as we hope to show next, when we take seriously these ideas of interests, belonging and attachment as both pointing to borders and actualizing relations of helping, then instances of negotiation or connection between family and formal care practices are not so much negotiations 'between free humans who must be ready to change as the situation changes' but rather negotiations that are always already constrained by the actualities wrought by diverging attachments and interests (Stengers, 2005a, p 193).

In short, through focusing on relationships of exchange at thresholds, we see formal systems offering help from outside this threshold. If a family can figure out how to make use of the help, they accept it – they enter into the exchange – and are sustained for a time. Eventually a time comes when what is offered as something to exchange at the border can no longer be figured as help – and sustaining can no longer hold – this is the limit of helpfulness. 'Help' may be actualized when a family's attachments and interests are properly addressed, and the point of non-helpfulness occurs at that moment when the constraints of belonging to a particular practice are either not recognized or (simply) cannot be accommodated by 'other' practices. But in each case, care for the borders calls for attending to the logic of the between, that is, recognizing that actions at thresholds, and connections made, are partial and precarious.

Ken and Marla: an interest in keeping up appearances

One of Ken's interests is in keeping up appearances and keeping everyday life as "normal" as possible, as much like life "before" as possible. Although the specificities of this have changed over time, this interest maintains a 'tensional traction' in holding Ken and Marla's day-to-day life together (Cooper and Law, 2016, p 208). For example, in the beginning Ken and Marla made efforts to stay in touch with friends, and Marla had been continuing to visit with her 'sorority sisters' up until about a year ago. But over time, slowly, Marla was no longer able or willing to keep up with all of the activities they used to do on a regular basis, friend gatherings, theatre outings and all of the other events they are invited to. Everyday responsibilities have shifted, too, even while essential routines, like cooking and eating meals together, are maintained. As Ken says, "in fact it used to be my job to set the table while she did the cooking and then it got to be okay, I'll do the cooking, you set the table." But that also got to be too complicated and confusing for Marla, so now when Ken is cooking, he just tries to keep Marla out of the kitchen – "I've had to put stools across here just to keep her out" (Field notes, September 2015).

Ken shows his interest in keeping up appearances in other ways as well – for instance, in his efforts to help Marla choose clothes, to keep her teeth clean and her hair brushed. Even though these activities have gradually become a lot of work, maintaining norms of appearance and behaviour remain important – especially, it seems, as Marla has become less interested. Maintaining routines even as they change, and helping Marla remain in line with the appearances both of them have worked to present to the world over the course of their married life, are ways that Ken also marks Marla's decline. As Marla's ability to keep up appearances wanes, and becomes something Ken needs help with, outside help is sought. Ken writes to the doctor, asking the physician to explain the changes they are experiencing in order to help Ken account for what Marla can and can no longer do (see Chapter 6). It is as though Ken requires the doctor to take the lead on this, not only to legitimize and confirm Ken's observations, but also to help him to link Marla's changing capacities to keep up appearances to her illness rather than to any other reason.

From the outside, it could look like all this work of keeping up appearances is not worth the trouble it brings, but at the same time, it is important to recognize that Ken's interest in keeping up appearances is in no sense superficial. From the inside, it could be that keeping up appearances is also keeping their life together, keeping their history together as a married couple intact. For instance, despite Marla's incontinence, Ken and Marla continue to share a room and a bed. Ken talks about this in a matter of fact way one day, in the course of talking about how concerned he is with Marla's hygiene:

FIELD NOTES

September 2015

Ken tells me that getting Marla to put her head under the shower, even though it was a struggle, was really so she could get soap off her face and especially in her private parts – [cleanliness] was really getting to be a big issue and somewhere along the line, he's not sure exactly when, she started wetting her regular panties often enough, including soaking the bed one night. He says 'I ended up with her in Always Depends [incontinence pads], which help, but a couple times even, well several times now, she's flooded them even though they were dry when I put her to bed and I get her to go to the bathroom

before, sometimes she floods them at night and they've overflowed.
So now we have a waterproof mattress under the sheet'.

As noted earlier, this interest in keeping up appearances, maintaining a sense of "normal" life, is a lot of work, but it also seems critical to the family practice. What helps Ken and Marla with this? What are the "bits and pieces" that are helping Ken and Marla with keeping up appearances and thus keeping their lives together? Certainly having Marla enrolled in a day programme is a help. However, knowing he has to take her to the day programme means that Ken has a good deal of work to do to help Marla look presentable at the programme, but this seems to be offset by the opportunity, for both of them, to get out of the house and to be with other people. Knowing about the phases of dementia as set out in helpful materials Ken has picked up from the physician's office as well as from the support group he has attended also seems to help. His knowledge of the dementia trajectory means that he can align Marla's behaviours with sequential phases of illness progression. For example, as we described in Chapter 6, Ken writes about his concern that Marla may have an 'auditory processing disorder', something he has read about as a sign of progression of dementia. When Marla does not follow even simple instructions, this can be read as a sign of the disease and not intentional resistance – to him, to cherished aspects of their lives together – on her part.

Over the course of time that Ken cares for Marla at home, a case manager offers help of varying sorts. Something that Ken says is helpful is the presence of a healthcare aide assigned to Ken and Marla for a few hours each week, although how this is helpful also changes over time. For example, Ken talks of how in the beginning one of the care aides helped Marla to pick out her favourite Christmas ornaments, and how he asked her, and she was able, to help Marla bake her traditional Christmas cake (Field notes, September 2015). So initially much of the care aide's time was spent helping Ken and Marla to "keep up appearances", to engage in everyday, enjoyable and "normal" activities – walks outside, baking cookies, and looking at old photo albums. But over time these pleasant activities are gradually replaced with the work of personal hygiene for Marla, a different mode, but still the same interest, of keeping up appearances. As Ken says, "so now when [the home care aide] comes over, there's no activity, and all the colouring and any other kinds of things that they've tried to do has gone away" (Field notes, September 2015). But even so, the care aide is a critical element of the "bits and pieces" holding everyday life together, but importantly it is not just any person, it is Carole:

FIELD NOTES
September 2015

I arrive as planned, but it takes some time for Ken to come to the door – he has forgotten I am coming today. But it's okay he says, Carole is here [the home care aide] and the three of them were just settling in to watch some old vacation videos. Carole has been a regular home care aide with Ken and Marla for about three months. She tells me that at first they used to go for walks but now things [that is, showers] take longer, and that's what she focuses on. They used to play games, and according to Carole, Marla had more energy and alertness so it was easier to fill up the time. I ask what she does to make the work easier now – she says 'It is important to know your client and their routines.' ... Her tasks, she says, can include meal preparation, socialization and hygiene – she has tried over the months to keep Marla involved in simple household tasks like laundry or dishes. But she notices 'a lot more confusion now' – she and Ken tell the story together, lots of eye contact between them and head nods. She observes about the changes in Marla – 'seeing the changes [over the three months], she's totally different, it's crazy'.

What seems clear in this encounter is that it is Carole, not a generic 'home care aide', who is partially and transitorily part of the family arrangements, and the logic of the relations formed in this 'between' location is helping these arrangements to be sustained. The relation is flexible, a collaborative practice of trying out different ways of accomplishing what needs to be done – they 'used to' do things one way, and now they are trying other ways. And it is very time-limited – a few hours a week. But it is helpful, in part, at least, because the helping actions 'fit' with Ken's interests of keeping Marla in the day-to-day "normal" – going for walks, engaging in household tasks and keeping clean. So while Carole talks about her work in one way, a discourse of formal care provision ("It is important to know your client and their routines"), the style of her practice enables connections over time that work to sustain the interests of Ken and Marla.

Home care aides coming into the home to relieve a spouse of the full responsibility of caregiving duties represents a common form of help offered by the formal care system, but these forms of help are not always experienced as "helpful" by families. Just briefly and by way of contrast, the Cruz family was also offered and accepted this kind of help:

FIELD NOTES

July 2016

Katherine tells me that home care is coming to the house now, this was started last month. Someone comes Monday and Friday to help David shower, and Wednesdays for 'grooming'. I ask if this is helpful – she says 'it helps me a little bit' – a problem has been that David does 'not clean up after a bowel movement' – and sometimes he was 'smelly'. It doesn't appear that anyone in the family has actively or physically undertaken hygiene for David – they have told me and the geriatrician that he is 'independent', that is, Josh mentioned that they tell David to go take a shower and then leave it to him to do. I ask Katherine if she stays around or goes out when home care comes – she says it is only one hour, so she goes downstairs to 'let me hide'.

Here, prior family arrangements tell something about how the household and family life has been organized around norms of privacy, an interest that has outweighed norms of cleanliness. Help is now accepted, but the interest in privacy around personal care for David does not end even when someone else comes in to perform it – Katherine 'hides' downstairs. Help is brought into the family arrangements, and acknowledged as in some sense helpful, but at the same time it seems to 'conflict or wound' (Starobinski, 1975, p 342) rather than 'fit' with the Cruz family's practices.

To return to Ken and Marla, while Carole's visits are experienced as helpful by Ken, the time that the home care aide is assigned to them represents only a small fraction of all of the hours Ken is responsible for caring for Marla. Marla's attendance at the day programme, another common form of help, while of longer duration takes up only another small fraction of the week. Day programmes are offered in this case, not with any direct interest in helping Ken keep up appearances but rather, to meet the health system interest in 'sustaining' Ken as a family caregiver in his home. These strategies offer Ken help in the form of release from the full-time responsibilities of caring for Marla for short periods of time. During the times that the care aide is present, he can leave the house to pay bills and perhaps even meet friends he would not otherwise see. This is a similar release that Ken is afforded when Marla is at the day programme. But when each period of time concludes, Ken is pulled back into his role as primary caregiver, working hard to keep relating to Marla as his wife in order to maintain their life together, but watching her drift further into being the physician's patient (see also Chapter 6).

This becomes very hard work for Ken. He tells the physician at one of the last appointments he has in the Seniors Clinic that he is exhausted and is unsure if he can continue to care for Marla at home. He feels trapped. His calculation of all the hours when he is solely responsible for Marla transforms her as someone no longer able to participate as his wife. She does not talk to him. She does not respond when he asks her to do things. He tells the doctor that he has inquired into the possibility of having Marla admitted to a respite facility for just a few days. He thinks this would help him continue in his role as Marla's home-based caregiver. But a problem is that his case manager has told him that this sort of prolonged opportunity of having Marla cared for outside their home is not available currently, and will likely not be available for many months. Learning this has made Ken feel even more trapped. The physician offers medication that she says will help with Marla's compliance. She tells Ken it would "release" his "time to get things done by about an hour a day" (Field notes, September 2015). In offering this medication, the physician introduces her idea that Ken's trouble is that he is too busy with Marla to get things done at home. The medication would give Ken "an hour a day" that he currently does not have. But Ken's response to this suggestion shows surfaces that do not quite touch – Ken is feeling trapped in his home, and an extra hour a day is not going to help with that.

One outcome of this appointment is that Marla will be reclassified as requiring a level of care that now makes her eligible for long-term care placement. Prior to this her care needs had been assessed as suitable for a supportive housing situation, and this is what Ken had been hoping for, that Marla's first step out of their home would be to this kind of interim setting. But at present the wait list for supportive housing, like the wait list for respite placement, is very long. The waiting time for long-term care is much shorter, and Marla's placement will be prioritized. Marla's move to that home, to become the primary responsibility of staff there, all happens very quickly.

Everyone involved here has a common interest in sustaining this family, this arrangement of care, but in this particular 'zone of exchange' at the border between family and formal care practices, action and exchange of 'help' is being constituted by different interests and quite different sorts of knowledge. Ken has brought Marla to the appointment with the physician in an effort to demonstrate the challenges he is facing. Marla no longer speaks intelligibly to Ken. Ken is no longer able to engage her in even simple activities; they are alone in their home almost all of the time – what can be done? The physician's first response – offering medication that will alter Marla's behaviour, making her more compliant for a period of time during the day – does not match Ken's problem, it is not 'help' he can make use of. In this particular border exchange, the 'action' at the border does not seem to help; what is exchanged is an offer of help that does not meet what Ken seeks *as* help.

The interests of formal care providers in sustaining this family through the duration of the 'dementia trajectory' are realized through strategies such as offering a few hours from a care aide, a few hours in a day programme and the possibility of medication to reduce the demands on Ken. This is an idea of help as 'ready-made' – to put services in place, to add a few hours for help with a shower, to offer medication, all intended to help sustain the family, and to a certain extent this has helped. Some of the help offered, to become 'help', has been reconfigured – the few hours a week for personal care has become Carole with whom they have a relationship. She aligns with the family interests and for a time helps to sustain the arrangements. But now Ken has reached this point of feeling trapped inside his home. The inability of the physician to offer a response in exchange for Ken's 'problem' of being trapped marks what appears to be the limits of helping this family. Their interests have diverged to a significant extent, even though Ken maintains an interest in continuing to have Marla with him at home – he just needs a break. The points of connection here are very few. Stengers' (2019, p 190) question of 'who is, or will be affected, and how?' comes into sharp relief at this point, and it is not answered in this case in a way that can sustain the family arrangements. At this instance, in this moment, it is Ken's interests in keeping their life together that must shift. It seems there is nothing more to be offered as help that could cross the threshold that would enable Marla to continue to belong at home.

Colleen and James: an interest in being prepared

One of Colleen's interests is to "be prepared", and a key element of her care practice is to assemble the "bits and pieces" that might support this. In this way, gathering information is very important to her and she draws into the family arrangements information about how things with James are going to progress, how quickly they might progress and how she needed to position herself to be ready as the situation changed. Colleen understands the wider system of dementia care, that which takes place in people's homes, in hospitals and in long-term care homes. She understands that without proper planning, people with dementia can end up in hospital awaiting placement for many months, and they are there without programmes. She wants to ensure that this does not happen to James, and she knows that she needs to stay on top of things to ensure such unwanted outcomes do not come to pass. As part of her work of gathering information to be prepared, she has actively sought out people working in the community health system such as those associated with 'transition services'. After James has been assessed by a case manager and deemed to be someone who will likely, in the future, be placed in a residential care setting, Colleen starts considering possible placement sites. She tours some of these sites, checking on their relative quality with others she knows.

Throughout the time that Colleen cared for James at home, she was always on the look-out for information that she could bring home to help her in her caregiving duties. She had taken courses offered by advocacy agencies such as the Alzheimer's Association. These courses provided useful technical information that Colleen could use to keep her positioned as someone very well informed when she would meet with healthcare professionals. The information Colleen gleaned from print materials, organized neatly for easy retrieval from her binders, as well as information shared by experts in the field during courses designed for people caring for someone with dementia at home, was central to how Colleen conceived of help. These forms of help were helpful because they aligned with Colleen's interest in being prepared.

Just briefly, and again by way of contrast, "information", although a frequent form of help offered to families, is not always experienced as helpful:

FIELD NOTES

May 2016

Katherine tells me she has also been going to the 'Seeds of Hope' sessions that the Alzheimer's Society present – she has been attending the middle stage Alzheimer's session – she moves to the other side of the kitchen island to get the binder they have given her to show me the topics they have discussed. She finds it somewhat 'too much' – all the information she has been collecting or been given, from the Parkinson's groups, from the Alzheimer's Society, from home care.

But for Colleen, all this information can be made use of. Knowing what the healthcare system consists of meant, for example, that she could request access to as much external help and support as she and James were eligible for. She was introduced to the idea quite early on that she and James, in their 60s, were relatively young to be seeking access to community health supports. However, because Colleen had used the knowledge available to her and had pushed to have James diagnosed with dementia, they were assigned a case manager. Colleen developed a very positive relationship with their case manager. The case manager helped in bringing information into the home as well as sharing information about resources available in the community that Colleen and James could go out to benefit from. A healthcare system's interests in sustaining people with dementia in their homes for as long as possible prior to transfer into more expensive (for the healthcare system) residential care are different from Colleen's particular interests in having the information she needs to continue to look after James at home. However, their diverging interests need one another here to accomplish their common interest in monitoring and managing James' 'dementia trajectory'.

Safety was a key topic of discussion within the family as well as across the threshold of the home. While James denied that his cognitive ability was changing at all, Colleen and other members of the family became aware that he was having trouble finding his way to new destinations. Addressing this issue of keeping James safe from wandering and getting lost, including having him not continue to drive when it was determined that he was no longer responding appropriately to traffic cues, raised other safety issues in the home. The family's efforts to stop James from driving resulted in conflict between James and Colleen. Indeed, as Colleen and James negotiated through this period where Colleen felt she needed to determine how their lives together would proceed, she experienced James' behaviour as changeable and sometimes aggressive towards her. Rather than stepping back to reduce the likelihood of James becoming angry and lashing out physically, she set up events intended to push James to his limits. These experiments were encouraged, and sometimes participated in by healthcare professionals and were designed to help Colleen know better what James' limits were so that she could manage their lives within those limits. Here is just one example when an occupational therapist came to the house:

FIELD NOTES

April 2015

The occupational therapist [OT] arrives and comes up into the kitchen. James seems comfortable, displaying little curiosity, continues to eat his fruit. Almost immediately after sitting, and saying hello, she starts a series of rapid-fire questions in response to his questions. She speaks very clearly and loudly to him, with a somewhat exaggerated cadence, that is, like she might speak to a child. The questions are detailed, often in response to something he asked her; she turns it into a game but keeps pushing him to retrieve more information in response to questions. Sometimes James turns to Colleen to confirm an answer, but she refuses. Sometimes his stories in response to questions are confused or don't make much clear sense. Sometimes when the OT pushes, he goes back to what he knows. Then she stops for a while to let him finish eating.

So trying to achieve knowledge of James' limits gave Colleen something to actively work on, providing more information that she found helpful as she tried to maintain relationships with family and friends over time. This interest then, in being prepared, drives all the family's arrangements, entailing processes of adjustment and readjustment, bringing some things in and keeping other things out to keep everyday life on an even keel. But one problem was that James' limits were not always trustworthy, and that not everyone involved with James was concerned in the same way with knowledge of his limits.

When James was at his day programme, the staff there did not either have the knowledge that Colleen had or conduct the programme with that knowledge in mind – an instance, perhaps, of formal care systems offering help from "outside" but without recognizing this location as a relationship of exchange: Colleen's carefully assembled "bits and pieces" are not pulled into the action. Instead, despite Colleen's warnings about James' limits, staff permitted James and one of the other day programme participants to enter one another's space, and conflict with that person resulted. Initially, James raised his voice, signalling possible danger for the other person. Staff told Colleen about this incident and, drawing on her accumulated knowledge of James' limits, she advised that conflict could be avoided if James and the other person were kept apart. When monitoring of James' behaviour at the day programme again broke down, he and the other person became engaged in a physical altercation. The impact of the day programme's inability to learn from Colleen quickly became Colleen's problem to deal with. Despite being advised by Colleen that aggressive behaviours between James and the other programme participant could happen, staff decided that it was James who could no longer be trusted to attend the programme, and he was discharged. So a failure of a relation of exchange at this border resulted in something decidedly unhelpful, and as actions meant to 'help' sustain a situation come to be experienced this way, questions about the ability of the family member with dementia to remain, or belong, at home are foregrounded.

James' sudden discharge from the programme precipitated a crisis for Colleen, representing a marked breakdown in helpfulness between her and those representatives of the formal care system that she had cultivated good relations with over several years. For Colleen, the border of helpfulness came in the form of a well-organized week with James involved in routine activities inside or outside of the home, but in ways that meant Colleen could plan her own time accordingly. The programme had been very helpful to her and to James. It was not only the programme, but also its regularity, its dependability and the possibility it allowed for Colleen and James to spend time apart, thus decreasing friction between them. This was helpful for both James and Colleen. And that helpfulness sustained them for quite some time, until the sudden discharge, and then it no longer sustains the care arrangement.

If we examine relationships at this particular threshold, what seems notable is the lack of exchange, almost as if there is no recognition of an 'in-between' place, a threshold that actually requires the making of relations. While James was enrolled in the day programme, Colleen could operate on a dementia trajectory that left her with a good sense of control in relation to both her own and James' safety. Discharge from the day programme suddenly transforms the day programme from a mutually agreed plan for his care, an interest shared with Colleen, to simply a tactic used by the formal care system to sustain Colleen as the person responsible for caring for James at home. Here, the day programme is figured as a kind of 'container' for James, to be used for some part of each week, and when he can apparently no longer be contained there, he is simply released. But the day programme isn't only or essentially a container for James; it is a central part of the family's arrangements, it addressed their interests in being prepared and managing limits, and was thus necessary to enable them to 'go on', to be sustained at home.

Confronted with James' sudden discharge from the day programme illustrates to Colleen a significant breach in relations she has come to rely on in her work of caring for James. The zone of exchange at the border of helpfulness is revealed as inadequate, and importantly for Colleen's interest in being prepared, it is unpredictable. With James' participation at the day programme now suspended, Colleen can no longer see a way for her to sustain James on a dementia trajectory at home. If we think again about this question of who is affected and how by this course of events, this non-connection event at the border between family arrangements and formal care practices accelerates James' move to a long-term care setting – when daily life becomes too unpredictable for this family, it comes apart.

Katherine, David, Josh and Brent: an interest in maintaining a family as a family

It takes a lot of work and planning for the Cruz family to live together as a family in their home. We have described previously that Katherine and David live in a split-level home, and their sons, Josh and Brent, live with them. Four adults in this home where each level contains different and important parts of their life together: the kitchen on one level, a family room on another, bedrooms and bathrooms on another. As David's life with Parkinson's disease and dementia has progressed, more people and more things come into the home. While in some ways helpful to the family as they care for David, space for living everyday life seems to be getting crowded out. That the space for maintaining the family as a family is getting smaller seemed particularly visible during one visit in late November:

FIELD NOTES

November 2016

I arrive at the house shortly before 1 pm. As I am parking, I see a young woman walking up the driveway towards the house. I knock on the front door and enter, Katherine is greeting the young woman – I introduce myself to her, and say I am a researcher following the family – she is interested in my research, and says she thinks it's great as more needs to be 'done' for families. I ask if she is the physiotherapist expected; she says she is a physiotherapy aide (PTA) – she has come to show the home care aide (HCA) how to do some exercises with David. The physiotherapist has seen David at least once and has set out a programme for them to follow. Shortly after this exchange, the front door opens and a man in his late 20s arrives – this is Anthony, the HCA. Anthony is here from 1–4 for 'respite' – the PTA is going to show him how to do the physio exercises.

The division of labour among these members of the healthcare team introduces new people, each with a discrete task, into the Cruz's home. All these helpers bring items with them as they enter the home: shoes, papers, binders, pamphlets, pieces of specialized equipment. All of this adds to the already full home, and it also serves to separate the everyday work of caring for David that members of the family are involved in as they live alongside him from the specialized work that these professional caregivers provide as they come and go. All the attention also separates David out from the family – shifting him again and further from his identity as husband and father to that of identified patient. From the outside, this all looks like help to keep David safe; from the inside there is a question of how to sustain life together as a family in the midst of all these activities.

During the course of the afternoon, while information about the exercises is shared between the PTA and HCA, Katherine moves in and out of the bedroom where the PTA and HCA are working with David. The PTA has asked Katherine to purchase some specialized equipment for David to support him in getting around their home:

FIELD NOTES

November 2016

The PTA is looking for a 'transfer belt' and calls down to Katherine – she says she 'just bought one' and the PTA goes out of the room to get it. I hear them talking in the hall – the PTA notices David has a new walker [walking frame] and Katherine explains she just bought it. It then emerges that David's other walker broke 'the last time he fell down.' The PTA expresses concern and wants to know the details – 'When did he fall? Does the case manager know?' Katherine says he fell last Friday (four days ago) and says the case manager doesn't know. 'I'll tell her' says the PTA. Katherine explains she does not know exactly when he fell, 'I was sleeping.' The PTA asks 'Was he okay, did he get up on his own?' Katherine says she helped him.

The PTA's overriding interest in David's safety is unsurprising given David's tendency to fall and her particular role in healthcare, but it is not the same interest that Katherine enacts as she takes care of the equipment related to David's mobility – replacing the broken walking frame, buying a transfer belt for the physio to use – and helping him up when he needs help. Katherine doesn't 'report' the fall. Rather, in her everyday care practices, she just takes care of David when he does fall and tries to do things in ways that might help him avoid falling. But by telling the PTA, the information will now travel to the case manager, for what purpose it is not clear, especially as the impracticality of 24-hour-a-day supervision for David, as a way to prevent falls, emerges once again. But on this issue, the PTA has an offer of 'help':

FIELD NOTES

November 2016

Katherine starts to describe another, what she calls an 'incident' – when the PTA looks at her she says, he 'peed in his pants'. The PTA asks 'Can he not make it to the bathroom? Does he sleep in this bed? Would you try a bedside commode? The agency would clear it and send someone to clean it.' Katherine doesn't respond, she looks at the area by the bed and says that the space is too tight for a commode. The PTA says 'Hmmmm'. The falling is of concern to the PTA; for Katherine it seems part of their everyday. Katherine has gone back downstairs.

It now becomes relevant that David fell in the bathroom, and the PTA is suggesting bringing in a commode to the bedroom would perhaps stop the falls in the bathroom. The fall seems to be a signal to bring in more resources – more equipment – she will get her physio to reassess him – maybe, she says. Bringing in a commode seems to be suggested as a common practice – the home care agency apparently has arrangements in place to have people come to the home to specifically clean it. But Katherine is not going along – the space is too tight, she says, it wouldn't fit. Certainly a commode in the bedroom turns the home into something more institutional. But this is not Katherine's thinking; rather, her concern is something more practical. After the PTA leaves, Katherine says she doesn't want a commode in their bedroom "because when he goes to the bathroom, he often pees on the floor, it's messy, but there is tile in the bathroom and it is not too bad to clean up" (Field notes, November 2016). Meanwhile, the PTA is continuing to think of more ways to keep David safe:

FIELD NOTES

November 2016

'Maybe David should have someone walk with him all the time' she says. I ask her how she thinks the family might manage that (having someone with him all the time). She shrugs, and says 'The agency can bring in more help and I will teach Katherine how to do transfers.' Downstairs I can hear Katherine and her son, Josh, talking. She is talking about the new walker [walking frame]. I hear him say, 'Well, what can we do?' Katherine asks him if he has had lunch.

There is a great deal of action evident in this visit – actions occurring in the present as well as in the past that now have new significance in the present. Relations between people, equipment and routines are also touching at surfaces where precarious connections are in the process of working out what is going to hold together to constitute help for David and his family. The PTA is worried about the number of falls that have been reported to her during this visit, but she also has good organizational knowledge of resources available that 'the agency' could bring into this home to help. Her initial thought was simply to recommend that someone – likely one of the family members – should be walking alongside David at all times now. This sort of recommendation signals her interpretation that David's condition is worsening and requiring additional supports around him, nearer to him, to keep him safe. When the question is asked about how this family might manage such additional time commitments, the PTA seems to add this consideration into her calculations and includes resources from 'the agency' into a package of help she can conceive of for David.

Katherine has perhaps recognized that it is the new walking frame that has set off this chain of action focused on bringing more care and assistance nearer to David as she speaks with her son downstairs in the kitchen, while also taking care of the more mundane task of lunch. Josh asks the rhetorical question in response to her comments about the walking frame, "Well, what can we do?" How to read this question? It could be that Josh is helping his mother recognize she had to explain to the PTA why David had a new walking frame and thus could not have avoided the further intrusion into their lives of the PTA and her concerns for David's safety. An alternative explanation for this question could be that Josh is commiserating with his mother, legitimately wondering what else can be done for David. It does seem that the relations between David and the home as it is currently configured, particularly when interests related to safety are made to drive practices, are increasingly problematic.

Even so, the PTA's suggestion of a commode at the side of the bed is not taken up by Katherine as helpful. The commode can be understood as a material object that the PTA has recommended be introduced into the home, but it is an object that enacts troublesome relations between the PTA and the family. The interests of the PTA in keeping David safe rub up against Katherine's interests in keeping her home going. Katherine's interests in maintaining her family as a family include a reluctance to add more foreign objects into her home (for example, the commode), but also all that the presence of the commode entails: the ability to keep the bedroom clean as well as the exposure of her sons to ever more intimate aspects of their father's care. It also keeps shifting the relations between Katherine and David away from their historical relation of wife and husband to Katherine being a caregiver for David. The rubbing up against one another of these interests, the tensions made between inside and outside, make it harder to know how to make use of the help being offered, how to incorporate it into the family's arrangements and thus make it helpful.

Reflecting on what such changes might mean for her after the PTA and HCA leave, Katherine says that she may well take up the suggestion made by the PTA to keep the case manager informed of David's falls:

FIELD NOTES

November 2016

Katherine says maybe she will call and ask for more 'respite'. 'It is better she knows there's more falling down in this house.' After a few minutes she says, 'People tell me to cut down on my volunteer work.' Currently she volunteers with different groups, probably several times per week. 'But I need it', she says.

Katherine signals in her comments something of how everyday life feels at this point on the dementia trajectory. She knows she can call the case manager for more assistance in caring for David – she could have a commode brought in, more respite hours – but it seems that it is difficult to know how to make use of the 'help' that is on offer, perhaps because this help is tied to the system's overriding interest to keep David from falling. The materials of helping don't fit so well with the interests of the family, which are concerned with safety but also with maintaining relations as a family who live together and help each other out, but who also have their own activities. Perhaps as an indication of the time she already commits to those activities of caring for David, she says that "people" tell her she could alter the balance of her commitments away from some of her outside volunteer work in order to free up time for David. But evidently volunteer work outside of her home is something necessary to Katherine – "I need it". Katherine is trying to continue defining in her own manner what matters to her, but all the "bits and pieces" at the threshold are telling her that "safety is most important" – and this becomes very hard to resist. And again, as Starobinski notes (1975, p 342), the contact surface between the inside and outside can be a place of exchange, but also the place of 'conflicts or wounds'. Katherine expresses her own 'conflicts and wounds'. Despite all the help offered across that border, at this moment, Katherine is feeling that "there is no hope", the help does not align with a possible future where the family is sustained as a family (Field notes, November 2016). Within six weeks, the family makes a decision in consultation with the case manager to have David transferred to a long-term care residence. The point of institutionalization comes when more 'help' doesn't help, when the situation, with all its moving parts, can no longer be sustained in a way that supports David to keep belonging at home.

'Addressing people as they belong': a challenge of borders

In one way, what we have tried to show in this chapter is what Latour (2007) describes as the 'thickness' of things. We try to learn about family care practices by giving a '*post hoc* narrative thick description of what should have been visible in the gathering' that holds and ties these practices together (Latour, 2007, p 142). Our descriptions represent an effort at making visible what has been there all along but is not always noticed. We have used this phrase 'belonging at home' through these sections to convey something of the wider sociomaterial relations (Cooper and Law, 2016) within which life with dementia and care at home for a person living with dementia is taking place. Such relations are not merely background or context, but are circumstances that are operative – part of the making things matter (Stengers, 2009).

Part of what we hoped to make more visible in showing what is gathered here are the ways that a family's care practices can be imagined to be activated by an interest in belonging – how to keep family members part of the everyday life of the family, how to materially and practically sustain their capacity to belong at home, part of a family's historical ways of living together. In illustrating the interests at play for families as they learn about how dementia is affecting their family member, we have also learned about a range of intricate and thoughtful practices enacted in the course of the days, nights, weeks, months and years of caring represented in these stories. The actions taken by families develop slowly and in line with their developing knowledge of their family member living with dementia. All of these careful, thoughtful, specific activities, designed to respond to the concerns of each day of living with a progressive disease like dementia, when examined as being in relation to the families that enact them, offer glimpses of those families' practices – they show to what that family is attached.

These intricate practices and the interests they reflect confer on each situation the power to matter in a particular, rather than a general, way (Stengers, 2005a). They describe problems that are particular problems for the people involved and the practices to which they belong. It is the singularity of both problems and practices that institute 'borders' at the figurative threshold of the home, that define a difference between each practice and its outside (Stengers, 2005a). And all those materials – people, objects, information – around and through which helpful practices from outside the family can approach and possibly enter to further sustain the family, must cross a border, and such border crossings entail, as Stengers suggests, 'the practical certainty of misunderstanding'

(2005a, p 189). To remark on this is only to recognize that there is no 'situation where you can take the place of the other, that is, where the borders can be explained away, for instance through the appeal to something in common, stronger than the divergence these borders signal' (2005a, p 189). Borders cannot be explained away.

It is the impossibility of substitution of interests and attachments that characterizes belonging to a practice, which, if we follow Stengers (2005a) here, is something different than merely being 'part' of a practice (as in we are all 'parts' of society). She writes of belonging in this way: 'Because of the fact I belong, I am able to do what I would not be able to do otherwise. In other words, addressing people as they belong means addressing them in the terms which Bruno Latour called "attachments"' (Stengers, 2005a, p 190). And it is this latter, thicker sense of belonging we wanted to explore in this chapter. It is why we have tried to understand borders, the divergent practices inside and outside these borders, the interests that form and reform them, and the relations of exchange in the spaces between – those spaces in which, in this chapter, we have located 'help'.

If, as Stengers (2005a, p 189) writes, 'where practices are concerned what comes first is the etho-ecological difference between a practice and its outside', how then to understand and manage the delicate operation of approaching to help? Here we look again to Stengers' (2015 [2009], p 143) idea of diplomacy that requires 'not a respect for differences but an honouring of divergences'. Honour, she writes, 'is something that will be apprehended not as a particularity of the other, but as what makes the other matter', that which cannot be reduced to the 'same' (2015 [2009], p 143). If we imagine approaching families to help with this idea of diplomatic practice in mind, divergence is made present and important, and not overlooked. Our address to families would need to be in and through, and in light of, their interests and attachments. Practices of helping would not be merely a matter of negotiation or goodwill, actions undertaken in spite of borders (Stengers, 2005a, 2015 [2009]). Negotiation, for example, always involves the shifting of borders to assure common interests ("safety is most important"), a give and take, a realignment or suppression of one of the parties' interests, a cajoling to just 'go along', to accommodate that more powerful, in some cases because it is needed, 'other' practice. As we have tried to show through this book, through our examples and stories, even when there seems to be common interests, for instance a shared interest in the 'dementia trajectory', these cannot be the same interests because the primary situation is one of divergence – divergence in ways of being, behaving and meeting the demands of the specific situation (Stengers, 2015 [2009]).

We know that practices of larger care systems are divergent as well, with distinct interests and goals. Representatives of these other practices, case managers, care aides, physiotherapists, and physicians may all have an interest in sustaining families; however, their practices are also attached to another set of practices largely aligned with the 'careful management' of expensive and limited resources (CIHI, 2017, p 27). For instance, the grammar of the 'dementia trajectory' can reflect, not a family's months and years of finding good ways to get through each day, but a kind of shorthand used to comprehend and manage the allocation of scarce resources – how many people are affected? When and where are they along this trajectory? What amount of 'help', and what timing, would mitigate effects on health and social care systems? Here the syntax of help can work as a strategy to prop up families. But this is a 'thin description' (Latour, 2007) and cannot possibly contain all the divergent, unique interests generating practices that are proper to the interests held by each family in sustaining themselves at home.

So, is the problem to worry about how to keep people with dementia out of the larger care system, to keep them at home? Or can we imagine a different challenge – how to support families as they travel along to a place where this person can no longer belong at home? There is always a limit of helpfulness, but perhaps 'help' could be reconfigured as a technology that might enable this belonging (Stengers, 2005a), rather than for any other reason. This might also accomplish the other interest of 'delaying institutionalization' but, in keeping borders and thus practices intact, how the limit of helpfulness gets reached could perhaps be less frequently wounding.

8

How to sustain a good life with dementia?

… an instruction is always a story cut too short.
Sravansky and Stengers, 'Relearning the art of paying
attention: A conversation', 2018

FIELD NOTES

September 2015

Wednesday is one of Marla's regular day programme days. Ken tells me that he has been unable to use DATS [Disability Action Transport Scheme] (the transport provided) because it is difficult to ensure that Marla will be ready to go on time – getting up and dressed is a struggle some days, and if Marla isn't ready, it's a problem. Plus, he was never sure exactly what time the van would arrive, and having her dressed for outside and waiting was an issue. I am going with them to the day programme because Ken thinks it is important for me to see what they do there and how important it is for him that she goes there (she now attends three days/week).

I arrive at the house at 8:40 – Ken has asked me to arrive early because he wants me to 'see' what getting ready to go out is like. I arrive, the house is very tidy, breakfast dishes have been washed and put away, radio is playing music, both Ken and Marla are dressed. Marla is wandering around the house.[…]

He finds Marla and says 'Let's go do your hair' and takes her into the bathroom. She resists his brushing her hair but then they decide she looks nice. He then helps her to brush her teeth and is concerned when she swallows the toothpaste; he tries to get her to rinse her mouth and admonishes her about the toothpaste. Then he tells her she 'looks good, really sharp'. He seems to go back and forth between gentleness and sharpness.[…]

Getting Marla into her outside jacket is a struggle. Ken tries to reason with her 'I just put it on, why take it off?' It's a chore to have her sit long enough to put her shoes on. Ken goes to get himself

ready to leave and I walk around the house with Marla. She says
'Ken is always fussing'.

In this excerpt Ken is showing a "normal" day, as if to ensure that it is
the practicalities of 'doing dementia' at home that become part of their
story. The goal of this particular visit was to see how things worked
at the day programme, so we could have just met there, but then the
work to comb Marla's hair and brush her teeth, to get her dressed for
outside, the adjustments to the car (a crib mattress on the seat in case
of incontinence) that are part of their current "doing" of dementia,
strategies that make possible their engagement in activities outside
their home, wouldn't have been 'seen'. So this could be thought of
as a kind of knowledge making in which dementia is shown to the
researcher as a practical problem rather than only something located
inside Marla's head. As Moser (2010, p 278) has shown in her work
on good dementia care in institutional settings in Norway, dementia
is something 'found in interactions and daily life', affecting most of all
how people live together, and in this context what is urgent is 'how
to make this life bearable, and preferably even pleasant and good,
here and now' (see also Thygesen and Moser, 2010). Ken and Marla's
here and now shows some of what is thought good, the continuing
relevance of social norms of appearance and behaviour, plus the work
of accomplishing these. Enacting these also brings trouble – Marla
resists, complains, undoes the work; Ken is alternately sharp and gentle.
There are some tensions here, goods and bads that need to be dealt with
together (Thygesen and Moser, 2010). And so we learn about Marla
as both a woman who can be helped to be (socially) presentable and
someone whose unruly bodily processes will be accommodated with a
crib mattress to protect the car seat. If we take these things and events
away, Marla is someone who can appear washed, brushed, dressed and
clean, as if independently, to be in the day programme – an appearance
that is reassuring. So this is a story that teaches about practicalities and
making these visible, and about how much effort, on both Ken and
Marla's part, is required to make a reassuring appearance, one able to
'fit' with social norms and expectations.

Part of what was surprising in beginning this study was the eagerness
with which the families involved chose to participate, their willingness
to share the details of their daily lives, to have them be seen. Many
cautioned us against adding to the "burden" of families' daily lives.
Yet, even as they worked to navigate and manage multiple activities,
including those of care, being involved in the research was treated by
families as something of value. Katherine, for example, from the midst

of all the family's various troubles, sent frequent email 'updates'. This one came before our plan to meet at the Seniors Clinic:

Hi Christine,
Before I will forget, the appointment will be on August 4th, 2:45. We will be picking up David from his day support programme around 2 then go to [X] Clinic. Lots of thing been happened:
Tuesday night July 16th, he fell face down, he had a cut in his nose and eyelid. We took him to the emergency room at [hospital]. The doctor sutured his nose. And told us to take him to the eye clinic at [hospital] the following morning at 8. Thanks be to God, it is only the eyelid that had a cut and one of the residents sutured it. They also found out that he has cataracts in both of his eyes. Follow up appointment will be this coming August 2nd with Dr X. We cancelled his dentist appointment that Wednesday. He was calm and didn't complain of pain. Antibiotics was prescribed.
Tuesday July 23rd, he fall again backward.
Wednesday, July 24th, dental appointment done, no issues.
With these falls he has been having lots of my friends and Josh told me that the trip to the [home country] is a NO and have a few suggestions that David needs a wheelchair since his right drop foot is getting worse.
A few incidents that when David pee, he miss the urinal.
Started this week, I added two more services so Monday and Friday it is a shower day, the rest is morning grooming. I felt so bad with my sons that have to undergo these things. We have our frustrations and I don't know how far can we take it?
I guess this is all for now
God bless!
Katherine (Email, July 2016)

Katherine reaches out with a list of events constituting an update about what's been going on – many of these seem to reference David's (failing) physicality – his falls, cut eyelid, now cataracts, cancelled dental appointments, wheelchairs and foot drop, incontinence and urinals, showers and morning grooming. What is it that Katherine wishes her sons did not have to undergo? In daily life the physical body is often taken for granted, unnoticed – but here it projects itself as something for others to 'undergo'. These are 'events' that Katherine tracks to show how they are now doing the disease, telling about a household increasingly organized around David, his care and safety, and about the trials of needing to be organized in this way – the difficulty of maintaining the 'norms' of family life, there are feelings that are bad, and frustrations, but even so, they somehow need to be shared and shown. And yet these events are not just 'feelings'; they are 'happenings', distributed and coordinated in material ways across the family, emergency services, home care support guidelines, numerous health professionals as well as urinals, walking frames and wheelchairs – circuits, as Cooper and Law (2016, p 201) might suggest, of 'contact and motion'. So much going on – and presented here by Katherine to the researcher as something to be known about and learned from.

But this list, in the ways lists do, leaves a lot out – we can only imagine the fearfulness for David of frequent falls, the stress and worry of multiple visits to the emergency department (A&E), the actual physical labour of helping David from place to place to place, the frustration of cleaning up missed urinals, the hard decision to breach family privacy norms and accept outside help. Katherine's list tames and contains this complexity (Mol and Law, 2002), allowing it to be passed along, much like the assessment provided somewhat later by a transition coordinator when the move to long-term care is being contemplated: 'We [Katherine and Chris] read what has been written so far in terms of the reason for assessment: "difficult for the family to manage", "falls, incontinence, feeding"' (Field notes, December 2016). As we [Katherine and Chris] discuss this assessment, and the reasons for it, what emerges is that this brief notation also tames and contains a lot of fear – fear they have given up and been given up on – as well as feelings of exhaustion and frustration, concerns about money and the costs of long-term care and most of all, worries about what will happen there, because Katherine has been told that 'once you put him in there, they go fast' (Field notes, December 2016). And even if it is the case that there are good reasons for the economical language practices of healthcare, there is still a question of, as Law (2004, p 2) argues, 'how might we catch some of the realities we are currently missing?' Law is most concerned with our characteristic research methods for knowing the social world, but there is a relevance here that we saw emerge in our discussions with formal care providers about this work (described in Chapter 3), a ruefulness captured in this comment from one participant in a provider group: "We assume that they can handle the burden and focus on task things, so we lose the other things that improve quality of life. We miss the whole picture of what does this really look like for the family and the person with dementia" (provider group). As with Katherine's email and the transition coordinator's summary, there are benefits to be associated with such seeming clarity, but as Law observes, 'simple clear descriptions don't work if what they are describing is not itself very coherent' (2004, p 2). So Katherine's email and the transition coordinator's notes can only gesture to a world not so coherent, raising questions about our practices of knowing and the kinds of worlds these practices may make, worlds that in being simplified in this way may come to seem more manageable than they actually are (see also Chapter 2). And if this thinking has merit, we will, as Law argues, 'need to think hard about our relations with whatever it is we know, and ask how far the processes of knowing it also bring it into being' (2004, p 5).

Helen sends a note shortly after Christmas asking if we should arrange a visit, 'just to catch up':

FIELD NOTES
January 2016

Albert opens the door for me, and smiles and says hello. I enter and we sit, as usual, at the kitchen table in the front room. I notice a bit of a pungent odour in the house – maybe from cooking, but it is difficult to identify. Albert and Helen are 'eyeing' each other – and Helen explains they've just been having a 'spat'. She tells me that they were supposed to go to the bank this morning, after she returned from meeting her friend for coffee – but the 'bank papers' were no longer where she had put them, and Albert denied moving them – they ended up searching all over the house to find them. She points them out to me on a shelf by the front door – there are about ten envelopes bound together with a rubber band. She says Albert should just leave things, and that there is too much paper in his office, and although he claims to be always able to find what he needs, they are always looking for things. Albert is not defensive, just shrugs off her annoyance.

Part of the problem, Helen says, is that 'he's always paid all the bills' – she wants to know how to do it but it is new for her … it seems Helen is gradually taking over the banking tasks, even if it means driving to the bank twice per month to deposit cheques and pay bills. She says she is comfortable with driving to the bank – she knows the route well and they only go during quiet times. They both share in giving me a detailed description of the location of the bank relative to their home, and how they get there, how they avoid a particular intersection because there is no traffic light.

This leads us into a conversation about driving in general, and I ask if Albert has been driving since the doctor told him not to. He says not and Helen says he's 'been really good'. ... I ask if Helen is a good driver. They agree she is, but then Helen describes some of her driving issues. For example, her 'side' vision is very bad, and she says 'I can't back up – so I get him to do it'. So he is still driving a little. She says she mostly feels 'safe' but doesn't like driving on one particular roadway (a multi-lane expressway) – so she just goes to the middle lane and stays there 'I feel safer in the middle' – other cars can go around her. Also, she says 'I can't see addresses, I never could' – so they only drive places they've been before. Helen adds she does not like to drive at night – partly because she can't see as well. It seems Albert helps with this as well, though how is not clear.

Albert and Helen are managing despite things going "missing", and despite occasional "spats" about this. A problem is that they're always looking for things, searching the house for needed papers such as the ones they needed to go to the bank. In this and in the discussion about driving they show the accommodations being made by both of them, the shifts in their relationship, new things brought it, the redistribution of daily work – although it also seems that these shifts are not settled, needing to be continually worked out and on. Albert used to do the banking, but now Helen is learning how to do that – but it means that sometimes Albert will move the papers that Helen needs. The driving question suggests the looseness of their daily accommodations. In a biomedical frame, it seems simple – in an earlier medical appointment, Albert has been told quite definitively that he should not drive and the doctor had emphasized that "driving is a medical issue and a public safety issue", supporting her position with reference to changes in Albert's MMSE – his "numbers" have gone down (Field notes, December 2015). In the appointment this was an instruction that everyone seemed to accept, or at least it went unchallenged – today, Helen and Albert would probably say they are adhering to it. But through listening to them talk in this visit it seems less clear – it emerges that Albert helps Helen with her driving – she has trouble backing up the car, so Albert does this. Together they plot out the best driving route to the bank, taking into account the weather, traffic lights, parking and time of day. They limit their destinations, and only go to places they've been before, and it seems they only make necessary trips, such as to the bank. It seems that they are using different knowledge than the doctor, who seemed to rely mainly on an individualistic measure of Albert's memory and cognition over time. What Helen and Albert demonstrate is different, a sort of combined or even perhaps multiplied knowledge that they do together. Their knowledge is of necessary tasks, different skill sets, complicated terrain and routes through it – and it is this knowledge that guides their daily management of transportation issues. On the one hand, they know they have to pay attention to the doctor's instructions; on the other, Helen can't back up the car or see well at night. So there is a sense that while the doctor's expert knowledge frames a key problem they confront on a day-to-day basis, with her work localizing the issue in Albert, their experience of living at home presents different problems so that what is actually done to make a day work draws on a somewhat different set of knowledge practices. The normativity that emerges from daily practice is one that tries to improve the situation, make it liveable for right now, rather than fix it once and for all; it relies on somewhat precarious workarounds rather than prescription, or laying down the law. They haven't ignored the doctor's injunction but have amended it slightly, made it more workable, or worked out in private what they, Helen, together with Albert, can live with. But it doesn't fit well with the seeming clarity attained during that doctor's visit, it doesn't seem like the same world at all. So this is a story that tells about the unsettledness of even that which appears to have been sorted.

And then there is Colleen who, from the first, deliberately ensured that what mattered to her, and what "helped" her, was visible in the research. She and James were dealing with a situation in which "control" was thought to be at stake, and so drawn into their arrangements were things that create (a sense of) control – binders full of information that will help plan the future, the searching for "missing pieces" and gathering together resources – knowledge about dementia and how to be a caregiver and how to use available system supports and how to draw others in – the case manager, the day programme staff, the geriatrician, her family doctor and even James' family. The work of managing this condition, and knowing about it and what can be done in relation to it, is distributed across the binders, notebooks, courses, other books she reads, people she talks with – since this can't be fixed, what needs to be done is manage it. She makes a massive effort to make something that works, this careful and capable woman, and then, despite all her efforts, in the end her work comes undone. Her practice, so similar to, perhaps even patterned after, the practices of formal care providers hadn't been able to account for parts of her plan giving way. Institutions are supposed to be stable and predictable, formal care providers are supposed to be there when you need them. And it is not so much to say her faith was misplaced but that the 'strong boundary' (Cooper and Law, 2016, p 201) of organizations turned out somewhat more insubstantial than she had imagined – despite the seeming solidness of their appearance in her binders, appointments and courses. Rather, what she confronts is 'more like assemblages of *organizings*', showing how organizations such as 'community-based healthcare delivery' 'are really *effects* created by a set of mediating, measuring instruments' (Cooper and Law, 2016, p 201; original emphasis). They are not so solid as they sometimes appear. This story also reminds us of Gronemeyer's (2017, pp 20–1) assertion that not only does 'dementia evade planning', but its ability to throw our best plans into disarray creates 'irritating tasks for the planning, rational, future-oriented modern society'.

'Trying to listen to that which insists'

It may seem a bit unusual in this final chapter to not come directly to a 'conclusion', to instead come at our ending sideways by telling a few more stories. But, as Tsing (2015, p 37) shows in her study of ecological life, 'to listen to and tell a rush of stories is a method', but as a method, stories 'have a problem with scale. A rush of stories cannot be neatly summed up'. Stories do not 'nest neatly'; they just keep interrupting (Tsing, 2015, p 37). Participant families' 'everyday' was the entry point for our study, attending to what people were doing, how they found ways to negotiate the demands placed on them, showing what they hoped to accomplish and the trade-offs they made in achieving this. These are storied experiences, what Tsing might call 'enabling entanglements', and as we have tried to show throughout the book, each story fosters a possibility of paying attention to different details, which makes details important to learn from, or, as Stengers suggests, in learning through details we could be provoked in our thinking (Savransky and Stengers, 2018).

In some part the provocation is simply constituted by the need to look, listen and learn, almost endlessly, about the practicalities, the events along with feelings they evoke and the actions they require, the continuing unsettledness of arrangements and the imperfection of plans. The provocation is understanding, being pushed to consider that if we want to 'help' in any of these situations, help would actually need to respond to the problem at hand – whatever that might be, and it would likely not be the same problem from one day to the next, from one family to the next. As a 'finding' of our study, this is not necessarily surprising or new, but it is provoking. And it is provoking in part at least, because it is not just the particulars of each family's practices that are shown in the details, but also the ways that family care practices are held together, and made to come apart, by the kinds of relations made with institutional routines, professional values and standards, biomedical practices and patternings, social ideologies of who exactly is responsible for care and how. In every story there are always the echoes and traces of 'other' practices, relations always in flux, and these have a lot to do with us and how we might know them. For Pols (2018), in her study of care and the everyday, the specificity of care, and we would add its changeability, raises questions about how to know it. Such specificity, writes Pols, 'raises the question of how to acknowledge the particularity of care practices and how to build an understanding of specificity into *the style of getting to know* these practices, in order to scrutinize and learn from differences rather than ignore them' (2018, p 59; emphasis added).

This question, we would argue, of 'getting to know' a family's practices is not only a question for researchers, but also a question for formal care providers who meet with families. And it is also a question for planners and policy-makers to take into account – there must be room, after all, in the plan to foster the kinds of relations that enable getting to know families' practices. As Law (2004, p 15), in writing of how to know the social suggests, 'we need to look at institutions if we are to create methods that are quieter and more generous' – a point we return to presently.

But why come to such an ambiguous place at the end of this book? To a large extent the troubles facing families cannot be 'fixed', but there is a question of whether and how they could be improved. Sometimes the little 'instructions' offered – don't drive, supervise 24/7, put a commode at the bedside, use your walking frame at all times, try this medication, avoid situations that antagonize, don't forget to "self-care", have a plan – while possibly necessary are also possibly not that helpful. They always seem to come up against a story that involves houses with stairs, bedrooms with carpet, day programmes with rules, constrained resources for "respite", not to mention each families' norms, values and routines as they engage in "muddling through" the necessaries of everyday living – continually relating to new situations, evaluating what needs to be done, adapting, accommodating that which has not been, and possibly cannot be, planned for. In the face of such stories, the instruction does not appear so helpful perhaps because, as Stengers (Savransky and Stengers, 2018, p 131) observes, 'an instruction is always a story cut too short'. The instruction, as it shows the limits of allowable concerns, becomes recognizable as an authoritative move, a powerful action that works to separate the 'concern' from the 'problematic path' through which it arose (Savransky and Stengers, p 131). It is however, this problematic path, and more, that marks the 'specificity' that Pols (2018) refers to earlier.

The formal care system, however, works with its own logics, values and standards of care. We saw this in our 'stakeholder' discussion groups (Chapter 3), in the vastly different responses to our film. The families who participated were unwilling to give advice or say what should be done, deferring instead to empathy for the ways in which 'it all goes back' to the family members to deal with. By contrast, saying what should be done seemed the first instinct of the provider groups, creating a sense of an orientation to the 'fix', to the instruction rather than the story. But an orientation to the 'fix' seems to bring along with it an often overwhelming rationality, articulating tensions between powerful ideas of planning and preparedness and the quieter, although no less insistent, question of for what would you prepare? And, as we saw in Chapter 2, it is not that 'dementia' as it figures in worries about population ageing or the costs and allocations of healthcare resources cannot be planned and prepared for, but these plans arrayed around 'system' preparedness do not show us what helps in a life lived with dementia.

It is for this reason that in this book we intended to try to offer an 'intervention' in thinking framed in terms of a different way to pay attention to what matters in everyday life in this context, to formulate the problem of care at home in a somewhat different register, and in so doing enable new questions to push through. We know the field of 'dementia care at home' research is pretty vast, and to some extent there is a 'known' storyline – that most care for people living with dementia is done at home, that this is care that comes with various challenges, that families seek help when it becomes too much, and that in times of economic restraint, options and resources for support are constrained. In this context we cast about for knowing what would be the 'best' thing to do only to find that there is no 'right way', no single solution that helps everyone – there is no ideal programme (see Chapter 2). The 'regularities and standardizations' we seek in striving to be 'helpful' have limits, no more so than when they try to impose themselves (Law, 2004, p 6; see also Ceci et al, 2013). It is trying to meet a world that is largely indeterminate, one that in its details often doesn't really have much of a pattern, that led us in the last three chapters to try to deepen and complexify our understanding of family care practices, and in this way to try to contribute to how to think about the situation we are trying to improve. This is not complication for its own sake, but rather, as Law (2004, p 2) argues, 'if the world is complex and messy, then at least some of the time we're going to have to give up on simplicities'.

It was Stengers' (2005a, 2005b, 2019) articulation of an ecology of practices that inspired us here. We had already located our work in terms of care practices studies (Mol et al, 2010), but Stengers pushed us to think through the implications of practices *among* practices which, as she argues, 'opens the question of what is proper to each practice' (Savransky and Stengers, 2018, p 137). Thinking through what is proper to each practice is part of how we thought to help establish a 'new practical identity' (Stengers, 2005a) for family practices, one that might shift relations between families and formal care providers in ways that might foster something like a relation of diplomacy. Such a relation would recognize that common interests, for example to 'delay institutionalization', are not necessarily the *same* interests, and would foreground that the challenging situation each party faces is not the same situation (Stengers, 2005a, 2005b). So, through Chapters 5 and 6 we showed that family 'care' emerges and is sustained through situated and singular practices that must also make relations with 'other' practices, specifically, a larger and quite powerful rational system of practices that sometimes 'helps' but also sometimes overwhelms. Throughout we see everyday practical arrangements and rearrangements, both the fragility and persistence of these, and we see that nothing is ever 'settled' once and for all; new solutions to new problems have to be found and this always implies risk – things may not work out. Chapter 7 showed practically what 'belonging' to a practice might mean in terms of enabling people living with a dementia to continue to 'belong' at home – and we see that though practices that enable belonging are similar to the project of 'delaying institutionalization', they are also completely different. It is this we have been trying to pay attention to, to learn from 'trying to listen to that which insists' (Stengers, 2009, p 19) as families shared and showed stories of their everyday lives.

So what can be done with what these families have tried to 'teach' us? An influential approach to concerns about population ageing and an increased prevalence in chronic conditions such as dementia is seen in an increasing focus on developing 'integrated' health systems. Integration is intended to create seamless and coordinated services for people, and to ensure that systems function more efficiently and effectively (Hollander and Prince, 2008; Hollander et al, 2009; MacAdam, 2009; Williams et al, 2009; Glimmerveen and Nies, 2015). While this is an important stream of research, the attention to 'system fixing' as a response to the growing number of older people underlines May's (2012) argument that management has become a central concern in chronic and debilitating conditions such as dementia. Here the problem for health and social care systems becomes not care per se, but the coordination of care as a way to optimize resources and manage demand – we heard the echoes of this agenda repeatedly in our conversations with key informants (Chapter 2) and from some of the 'stakeholder' groups who participated in our film discussions (Chapter 3). Integrating services, a response often assumed to enhance system 'navigation', is seen to support the shift of care to the home, and thus alleviate stressors that people living with dementia place on both institutional and acute health services, as well as smooth out the experiences of families themselves. But, as Mol (2002, p 182) points out, 'rationalization as an ideal starts from the idea that the problem with the quality of health care resides in the messiness of its practices', that is, a conviction that eliminating 'messiness' will somehow improve care. Instead, as we will suggest presently, it may rather be the case that some of these organizational care practices are not quite messy enough.

But before we turn to that discussion, we make the observation that while many involved in the provision of health and social care services acknowledge there are 'gaps' in the current system, it seems unlikely to us that such gaps are fully relatable to the question of integration. That is, in many respects the 'system' appears to be already 'integrated': it simply fails to include many of the care attributes that are important for people living with a dementia and their families (Nies et al, 2009; Liveng, 2011; Low et al, 2013; Tufte and Dahl, 2016). Much research, including our own (Ceci, 2006a, 2006b; Purkis et al, 2008; Ceci and Purkis, 2009), documents the gap between the kinds of help older people and families need and the kinds of services that a system such as home care tends to offer – both in terms of kind as well as level of service available (Health Council of Canada, 2012). In the case of dementia, such research suggests that families need flexible, responsive services able to respond to the unpredictability of everyday care needs – precisely the kinds of services rarely available in formal systems.

So an impasse of sorts and we are back again to our question of what can be done with what these families have tried to teach us.

'Embracing the messiness of the world'

In the absence of a 'cure' for 'dementia' and of a 'fix' for daily troubles, what constitutes goodness in care is open to question. And a question that needs to be asked when we think about this situation is whose problems are we trying to solve, and what knowledge is being used. To the latter point first, we know that family care practices in this context, and the knowledge embedded therein, have a quality of improvisation. The practical rationality of their daily lives demands this, skills of, as Pols (2010, p 419) argues, 'persistent solving of new puzzles and calculations with ever changing sets of variables'. The knowledge involved is highly contextual, focused on finding out how this particular situation, this here and now, can be understood and dealt with (Pols, 2014). The situation itself calls for improvisation rather than a plan to put into use, which makes it a rationality almost completely inverse to that of the logic evidenced in most health and social care delivery arrangements, although not completely, as sometimes we see something slightly different happening on the ground. We point here to an example from Chapter 2, specifically, the caregiver support therapist who, in thinking about how to put more 'care' around this problem of care at home, suggested the essential questions to ask are "How are you doing?", "Is it going okay?" and "What is the dilemma for the day?" These are 'small' questions that open the way to big worlds – not intrusive, not disruptive, but rather a style of getting to know a family (Pols, 2018) that seems to us to invite the possibility of improvisation, concerned with the here and now and how it may be improved. Such seemingly simple questions hold that quality of improvisation that might support people's local and practical attempts to improve daily life, envisaging a different kind of alliance between family and formal care. And echoing Stengers here, we don't know what difference such alliances would make, but we do think they would make a difference (Savransky and Stengers, 2018, p 137). A point, however, is that fostering such alliances needs a different set of practical conditions to enable the possibility of everyone involved being able to stay with, and work alongside, the 'messy' troubles and contingent specificities that characterize a family's daily life. It would require, as Law and colleagues (2013) might suggest, a system that does not try for purity so much. And while a 'plan' cannot necessarily 'contain' improvisation, it can certainly contain the space for it. It was in this context that we were drawn to consider Law and Mol's (1995) idea of patchwork. Conventional thinking would have patchwork in healthcare systems as a 'bad' thing, lacking organization, coordination, integration and coherence. But, as we asked in Chapter 2, when we see patchwork practices, is this evidence of system failure, or does patchwork operate as a kind of inclusive failsafe when conditions permit its operation? If control is what we are after, then yes, a patchworked practice can be seen as failure, but if creative improvisation is needed to meet families where they are at, then perhaps not. The patchwork option, although messy, potentially difficult to 'navigate' and likely difficult to manage, is also potentially generative. As Law and Mol describe it, to imagine patchwork is to imagine material and social – and stories too – are like bits of cloth that have been sewn together. It's to imagine there are many ways of sewing. It's to imagine there are many kinds of thread. It's to attend to the specifics of sewing and thread. It's to attend to the local links. And it's to remember that a heap of pieces of cloth can be turned into a whole variety of patchworks. By dint of local sewing. (1995, p 290)

It seems likely that to some extent at least, 'patchwork' may often be the character of the everyday practices of many formal care practitioners, and the point may simply be that this could be better supported. This seems important because, as Moser (2011, p 715) has argued, 'knowledge practices in health care are performative practices', the actions, frames of reference, routines and tools of practitioners and the organizations they are connected to do not merely statically address the also presumed static objects of practice. Rather, such knowledge practices also actively enact people living with a dementia and their families 'into being in particular ways' (Moser, 2011, p 715; see also Mol, 2002). In this view, we see that what is done, and what is thought should or could be done, in day-to-day encounters with families, may have significant effects in constituting ways of living with dementia, in bringing into being relations that improve this daily life, or overlook its actual character. And if the unavoidable character of this daily life leans towards uncertainty, localness and sometimes precarity, practical attempts to help will need to be able to relate to this – not least in the style of getting know the situations we are trying to improve.

The potential generativity of the 'patchwork option' may simply lie in the possibility of a plurality of pathways. Davina Cooper (2001, 2014) explores the idea of social pathways in her analyses of how social change happens and can be sustained, particularly change that might be construed as an oppositional (that is, an alternative to dominant norms and patterning) practice. Cooper writes about 'networks and spaces that perform regular life' but in a different fashion than we might be accustomed to, and while her interest lies in 'conceptual utopias' tuned to the possibilities of 'other, better worlds', the overlap with our interests here lies in this idea of the altered possibilities that are produced when regular life is simply performed differently (2014, pp 2–3). Doing things differently can instantiate new pathways – although whether these become normalized is an open question, reflective of the ways the 'environment pressures and steers' action (2001, p 121), with the idea of environment referencing 'the (often contradictory) complex of discourses, rules, resource allocations, norms and practices which structure, without determining, pathways taken' (2001, p 131). Cooper explains her metaphor of social pathways partly through contrast with the idea of trajectory, which is something we have discussed quite a lot in this book. A trajectory as a way forward is flattened, imagined from above and imposed (2001, p 128). Pathways, by contrast, are constituted on the ground, through 'being walked and woven' (2001, p 128). The difference here is one of scale, where each 'route' 'reveals certain characteristics or phenomena while distorting or obscuring others' (2001, p 128). Trajectory discourse, as has been part of our argument in the book, maps and constructs pathways for others, and draws in concerns and interests – social, political, economic and medical – that may or may not be relevant or helpful to the paths walked and woven by families. The paths walked and woven by families, however, while also social (rather than individual) pathways, are developed by people finding their way in an environment that may still push in contradictory directions but at least enables the pull of alternatives. The implication, as Cooper argues, is that less unified, more contradictory environments may actually be of help: 'a messy environment can facilitate a range of pathways because none fit snugly into the landscape' (2001, p 143). This then becomes what Cooper describes as the 'dilemmatic' environment (2001, p 143) – if it isn't clear what to do or what is to be done, there is only the option to keep trying different possibilities. This framing articulates the quality of improvisation already evident in family care practices, and is perhaps what formal care practices might learn to emulate and make more room for in the organization of care.

Uneasy relations: planning for the 'unplannable'

We end with some reflections on policy, specifically, what an orientation to planning for the 'unplannable' might look like. Planning, in philosopher and scientist Ursula Franklin's (1999, p 61) sense of the word, draws on a simple definition, 'arranging beforehand'. In this simple definition she says, 'there are planners as well as plannees; there are those who plan and those who conform to what was arranged beforehand', also noting that 'it is much more fun to plan than it is to be subjected to the plans made by others' (1999, p 61). Planning originates, she further argues, in prescriptive technologies, concerned mainly with strategies that maximize gain, efficiency and effectiveness, a production model in which, in theory at least, everything that matters is controllable. If it turns out in practice that this control is somewhat illusory, it is assumed, implicitly or explicitly, that we simply have not yet firmly enough grasped all the pieces in play, and that turning attention to enhancements in knowledge, design or organization is the best way to achieve control of that which continues to elude us. Production models, she argues, have become 'society's major tool for structuring and restructuring, for stating what is do-able and what is not', whether or not such a model is appropriate to the task at hand (1999, p 62). A problem for Franklin is that those prescriptive technologies characteristic of, embedded in, and even appropriate to materials production have swept outward, seeding, claiming and distorting most other realms governing the shared frameworks of social life. We are steeped in such practices, and in 'such a milieu', says Franklin, 'it is easy to forget that not everything is plannable' (1999, p 63). But, as she observes, there is 'something comforting in a production model, everything seems in hand, nothing is left to chance' (1999, p 26). The downside, however, or what Franklin describes as the 'enormous social mortgage' of prescriptive technologies, is a 'culture of compliance' – we come to accept more and more that there is only one way, the right way, of doing a thing, a best practice to be scaled up, planned to maximize efficiency, and assumed to work almost everywhere (1999, p 23). This is a familiar planning practice defining many current healthcare research and policy initiatives but one, in tending to consider the local and situated context of care as somewhat irrelevant, that might be, in Franklin's words, 'a ticket to trouble' (1999, p 26). This is because, as Franklin argues, planning for the unplannable, all those sorts of situations that call for continual improvisation and adjustment, including most activities of daily living, needs schemes that are different in kind from those of the prescriptive technologies of production models. Possibilities for daily living, and caring for that, can carefully, thoughtfully be arranged for but not 'planned, coordinated and controlled in the way that prescriptive tasks must be' (Franklin, 1999, p 24).

We bring Franklin (1999) in to close our discussion here because she points so clearly to our problematic – one that is neither new nor unstudied, but which continues to challenge. Mainly we refer here to the frequently lamented distance between policy and practice, which we understand as articulating a space conditioned by the contradictory demands of dominant planning technologies employed to stabilize the pressing priorities of health and social care systems, and the less certain but equally demanding dilemmas of everyday living that waver and shift from one day to the next. Ethnographic case studies like ours critically analyse the distance between these two locations, showing something of how the actualities of daily life with dementia articulate with ideological, practical and programmatic discourses and practices developed elsewhere (see also Mol et al, 2010; Schillmeier, 2017). In our study, families' everyday lives were often, although not always, at odds with the kinds of practices and programmes planned elsewhere, requiring them to adapt and adjust to priorities not necessarily their own. But this is neither new nor surprising – as Walsh and her colleagues (2020, p 7) observe, 'care structures in most countries are still designed to suit the providers of care rather than individual needs'.

But alongside this concern, and perhaps even more worrying, were the ways that policy plans developed at a distance, as well as formal care programmes perhaps planned a little closer to home, had a part in modifying and transforming, and at times impinging on, the everyday realities that the families in our study were dealing with. There are perhaps benefits to the seeming clarity associated with, for example, the ideal programme described in Chapter 2, but the powerful ideas of planning and preparedness associated with such endeavours, not to mention the tremendous efforts required to bring people into line with the plan, create worlds that in being simplified in this way come to seem both more manageable and more similar than perhaps they really are (see also Chapter 3, as well as discussions of 'the dementia trajectory' in Chapter 6). But once the 'plan' is in place, and shows itself to be successful, at least in its own terms, it starts to, as Franklin observes, 'represent the best or even the only way to deal with a situation' (1999, p 44). Its 'success' draws in almost everyone and everything – directing knowledge, organizational and material resources, producing specific practices and a 'mindset' that is difficult to dislodge (1999, p 14). The plan simply comes to be seen and deployed as the most appropriate tool to the task at hand, diminishing resistance to a prescriptive ordering of people and relations in an effort to solve the 'problem' as it has been defined by the plan.

At the same time, however, care needs a plan, and as Freeman (2017, p 194) reminds us, 'if care is a good thing, if we want to be sure of it when and where it's needed and not just as it might happen to be available ... then it will require some policy framework or complement, whether formal or informal' – care needs a plan despite a 'radical difference' between the worlds of everyday care and the formal policy-making practices meant to support it (1999, p 196). For Freeman, this radical difference is constituted in part by a crucial difference in epistemological practices, differences in ways of getting to know what the problem is, in determining to what we will pay attention (see also Lloyd, 2012). The individual specific and contingent case is the problem for those 'in the field'; the abstract, generic category of 'people living with dementia' is the problem for policy plans, as he says, 'in the office' (Freeman, 2017, p 197) (see also Chapter 2). 'In the office', the specificity and concreteness of the individual case must be 'faded out', its ragged edges smoothed over, in order to be able to appear in the generic terms that seem required for policy-making when the desire is to plan what may be done for 'everyone' (Freeman, 2017, p 197). So this is one possible and familiar problem, policy practices that smooth out differences, and in so doing create 'generic' conditions for care for 'everyone' – even though that 'everyone' may be, more or less, an empty signifier.

Schillmeier (2017, p 57) also critiques policy that creates 'pre-given formats' for care in this way, suggesting care policy, to be actually helpful, must become more 'real' – meaning creating conditions in which the specificities of emerging situations might be accounted for. And it may be the case, as Freeman (2017, p 197) suggests, that 'in the field' this is what formal care practitioners, those who enact the knowledge of policy in their everyday practices and actions, strive for. Such practitioners may take policy made elsewhere and address it to 'the case' with which they are confronted; they may 'translate between worlds' (Freeman, 2017, p 197). And indeed, we saw glimpses of this in our study, from those formal care practitioners who, despite their passionate advocacy of the need for a 'plan' (see Chapter 3), were still able to see that the actually helpful question to ask a family was 'What is the problem today? What is today's dilemma?' A problem may be, however, their ability to actually respond to 'today's dilemma' given the constraints of the plan. As Schillmeier argues, shared policy rules are only 'beneficial if they allow practitioners to respond adequately to the unfolding issues of care practices' (2017, p 55).

Freeman (2017, p 196) offers one way to think how to do this: instead of thinking policy as the 'product' of a rational and rationalized planning process, we highlight its status as 'process', and specifically, as a 'process of bringing things into relation with one another, or of forming new relations between things'. This is a helpful and loose understanding of policy-making, one to which we would add that it matters what kind of things and what kind of relations are envisioned as needed to be brought together. Some kinds of relations, prescriptive ones, are perhaps not the most helpful for families. But being wary of prescriptive strategies does not mean we are suggesting we should throw up our hands and do nothing. We return briefly here to what we have learned from the families in the study for guidance on this point: that the everyday practicalities of 'doing dementia' need to be part of the policy story, that shifts in daily life are never 'settled' once and for all, and that if formal care practices are not going to miss the 'whole picture' of what is going on, we need to build an understanding of specificity and localness into our styles of getting to know families and supporting family practices and arrangements. If we think again about Franklin's (1999, p 63) definition of planning as 'arranging beforehand', but shift our concern from arranging what is to happen to a consideration of how it might happen, that is to say, if we focus on means as well as ends, we may start to identify the different 'schemes' needed to be in place to support care at home, schemes that don't surrender to randomness but respond to it. It is not surprising that such schemes describe a way of working – having time enough to engage, to understand emerging and changeable situations, having access to those resources that might help, and supporting outcomes shaped by those involved in the actual work. Planning for the unplannable is not a contradiction, then, but rather articulates an understanding of the conditions of possibility for care.

References

Afram, B., Verbeek, H., Bleijlevens, M. H. C., Challis, D., Leino-Kilpi, H., Karlsson, S., Soto, M.E., Renom-Guiteras, A., Saks, K., Zabalegui, A. and Hamers, J.P.H., on behalf of the RightTimePlaceCare consortium (2015) 'Predicting institutional long-term care admission in dementia: A mixed-methods study of informal caregivers' reports', *Journal of Advanced Nursing*, 71(6): 1351–62. doi:10.1111/jan.12479.

Alvesson, M. and Sandberg, J. (2013) *Constructing Research Questions: Doing Interesting Research*, London: SAGE Publications Ltd.

Alzheimer Europe (no date) *France – National Plans for Alzheimer and Related Diseases*. Available from: www.alzheimer-europe.org/Policy/National-Dementia-Strategies/France [accessed 6 September 2020].

Alzheimer Society of Canada (2016) *Prevalence and Monetary Costs of Dementia in Canada*, Toronto, ON. Available from: archive.alzheimer.ca/sites/default/files/files/national/statistics/prevalenceandcostsofdementia_en.pdf [accessed 15 June 2021].

Ares, N. (2016) 'Inviting emotional connections to ethnographic research', *Qualitative Inquiry*, 22(7): 600–5. doi:10.1177/1077800415622507.

Armstrong, D. (1982) 'The doctor–patient relationship: 1930–80', in P. Wright and A. Treacher (eds) *The Problem of Medical Knowledge: Examining the Social Construction of Medicine*, Edinburgh: Edinburgh University Press, pp 109–22.

Åsberg, C. and Lum, J. (2010) 'Picturizing the scattered ontologies of Alzheimer's disease: Towards a materialist feminist approach to visual technoscience studies', *European Journal of Women's Studies*, 17(4): 323–45. doi:10.1177/1350506810377695.

Askham, J., Briggs, K., Norman, I. and Redfern, S. (2007) 'Care at home for people with dementia: As in a total institution?', *Ageing & Society*, 27(1): 2–24.

Ballenger, J. F. (2017) 'Framing confusion: Dementia, society, and history', *AMA Journal of Ethics*, 19(7): 713–19. Available from: https://doi.org/10.1001/journalofethics.2017.19.7.mhst1-1707

Beard, R. (2016) *Living with Alzheimer's: Managing Memory Loss, Identity, and Illness*, New York, NY: NYU Press.

Beard, R. and Fox, P. (2008) 'Resisting social disenfranchisement: Negotiating collective identities and everyday life with memory loss', *Social Science & Medicine*, 66(7): 1509–20.

Berry, B. (2014) 'Minimizing confusion and disorientation: Cognitive support work in informal dementia caregiving', *Journal of Aging Studies*, 30: 121–30. Available from: https://doi.org/10.1016/j.jaging.2014.05.001

Björnsdóttir, K. (2002) 'From the state to the family: Reconfiguring the responsibility for long-term nursing care at home', *Nursing Inquiry*, 9(1): 3–11.

Björnsdóttir, K. (2009) 'The ethics and politics of home care', *International Journal of Nursing Studies*, 46(5): 732–39.

Bond, J. (1992) 'The politics of caregiving: The professionalisation of informal care', *Ageing & Society*, 12(1): 5–21.

Büscher, A., Astedt-Kurki, P., Paavilainen, E. and Schnepp, W. (2011) 'Negotiations about helpfulness – The relationship between formal and informal care in home care arrangements', *Scandinavian Journal of Caring Sciences*, 25(4): 706–15.

CAHS (Canadian Academy of Health Sciences) (2019) *Improving the Quality of Life and Care of Persons Living with Dementia and their Caregivers*, Ottawa, ON: The Expert Panel on Dementia Care in Canada, CAHS.

Carpentier, N. and Grenier, A. (2012) 'Successful linkages between formal and informal care systems: The mobilization of outside help by caregivers of persons with Alzheimer's disease', *Qualitative Health Research*, 22(10): 1330–44.

Ceci, C. (2006a) 'Impoverishment of practice: Analysis of effects of economic discourses in home care case management', *Canadian Journal of Nursing Leadership*, 19(1): 56–68.

Ceci, C. (2006b) ' "What she says she needs doesn't make a lot of sense": Practices of seeing in home care case management', *Nursing Philosophy*, 7(2): 90–9.

Ceci, C. and Purkis, M.E. (2009) 'Bridging gaps in risk discourse: Home care case management and client choices', *Sociology of Health and Illness*, 31(2): 201–14.

Ceci, C. and Purkis, M.E. (2011) 'Means without ends: Justifying supportive home care for frail older people in Canada, 1990–2010', *Sociology of Health & Illness*, 33(7): 1066–80.

Ceci, C. (Producer) and Brunelle, J. (Director) (2018) *Care Collectives: Reconsidering Care in the Community* [film]. Available from: www.ualberta.ca/nursing/research/research-units/care-practice-research-network

Ceci, C., Björnsdóttir, K. and Purkis, M. E. (eds) (2012) *Perspectives on Care at Home for Older People*, London: Routledge.

Ceci, C., Purkis, M.E. and Björnsdóttir, K. (2013) 'Theorizing accommodation in supportive home care for older people', *Journal of Aging Studies*, 27(1): 30–7.

Ceci, C., Pols, J. and Purkis, M.E. (2017) 'Privileging practices: Manifesto for "new nursing studies"', in T. Foth, D. Holmes, M. Hülsken-Giessler, S. Kreutzer and H. Remmers (eds) *Critical Approaches in Nursing Theory and Nursing Research: Implications for Nursing Practice*, Osnabrück: Vandenhoek & Ruprecht, pp 51–68.

Ceci, C., Symonds-Brown, H. and Judge, H. (2018a) 'Rethinking the assumptions of intervention research concerned with care at home for people with dementia', *Dementia*, 19(3): 861–77.

Ceci, C., Symonds-Brown, H. and Purkis, M.E. (2018b) 'Seeing the collective: Family arrangements for care at home for older people with dementia', *Ageing & Society*, 39(6): 1200–18.

Ceci, C., Moser, I. and Pols, J. (2020) 'The shifting arrangements we call home: Struggles in home making and maintaining in care for people with dementia', in B. Pasveer, O. Synnes and I. Moser (eds) *Ways of Home Making in Care for Later Life*, Singapore: Palgrave Macmillan, pp 293–312.

Chia, R. (1998) 'Introduction', in R. Cooper and R. Chia (eds) *In the Realm of Organization: Essays for Robert Cooper*, London: Routledge, pp 1–11.

Chow, S., Chow, R., Wan, A., Lam, H.R., Taylor, K., Bonin, K., Rowbottom, L., Lam, H., DeAngelis, C. and Herrmann, N. (2018) 'National dementia strategies: What should Canada learn?', *Canadian Geriatrics Journal*, 21(2): 173–209.

CIHI (Canadian Institute for Health Information) (2010) *Supporting Informal Caregivers: The Heart of Home Care*, Ottawa, ON. Available from: https://secure.cihi.ca/free_products/Caregiver_Distress_AIB_2010_EN.pdf [accessed 15 June 2021].

CIHI (2011) *Health Care in Canada, 2011: A Focus on Seniors and Aging*, Ottawa, ON. Available from: www.homecareontario.ca/docs/default-source/publications-mo/hcic_2011_seniors_report_en.pdf?sfvrsn=14 [accessed 15 June 2021].

CIHR (Canadian Institutes of Health Research) (2013) *Living Longer, Living Better: Canadian Institutes of Health Research, Institute of Aging, 2013–18 Strategic Plan*, Ottawa, ON. Available from: cihr-irsc.gc.ca/e/47179.html [accessed 15 June 2021].

CIHR (2017) *Seniors in Transition: Exploring Pathways Across the Care Continuum*, Ottawa, ON. Available from: www.cihi.ca/sites/default/files/document/seniors-in-transition-report-2017-en.pdf [accessed 15 June 2021].

Clarkson, P., Abendstern, M., Sutcliffe, C., Hughes, J. and Challis, D. (2012) 'The identification and detection of dementia and its correlates in a social services setting: Impact of a national policy in England', *Dementia*, 11(5): 617–32.

Cohen, L. (1998) *No Aging in India: Alzheimer's, the Bad Family and Other Modern Things*, Berkeley, CA: University of California Press.

Collier, S. and Lakoff, A. (2005) 'Regimes of living', in A. Ong and S. Collier (eds) *Global Assemblages: Technology, Politics and Ethics as Anthropological Problems*, Malden, MA: Blackwell Publishing, pp 22–39.

Cooper, D. (2001) 'Against the current: Social pathways and the pursuit of enduring change', *Feminist Legal Studies*, 9(2): 119–48.

Cooper, D. (2014) *Everyday Utopias: The Conceptual Life of Promising Spaces*, Durham, NC: Duke University Press.

Cooper, R. (1997) 'The visibility of social systems', *Sociological Review*, 44(1): 32–41.

Cooper, R. (2003) 'Primary and secondary thinking in social theory', *Journal of Classical Sociology*, 3(2): 145–72.

Cooper, R. and Law, J. (2016 [1995]) 'Organization: Distal and proximal views', in G. Burrell and M. Parker (eds) *For Robert Cooper: Collected Work*, New York, NY: Routledge, pp 199–235.

CPSI (Canadian Patient Safety Institute) (2013) *Safety in Home Care*. Available from: www.patientsafetyinstitute.ca [accessed 9 September 2020].

Dalmer, N.K. (2019) 'A logic of choice: Problematizing the documentary reality of Canadian aging in place policies', *Journal of Aging Studies*, 48: 40–9.

Da Roit, B. (2012) 'The Netherlands: The struggle between universalism and cost containment', *Health & Social Care in the Community*, 20(3): 228–37. doi:10.1111/j.1365-2524.2011.01050.x.

Davis, D.H.J. (2004) 'Dementia: Sociological and philosophical constructions', *Social Science & Medicine*, 58(2): 369–78. doi:10.1016/S0277-9536(03)00202-8.

de la Cuesta, C. (2005) 'The craft of care: Family care of relatives with advanced dementia', *Qualitative Health Research*, 15(7): 881–96.

de la Cuesta-Benjumea, C. (2010) 'The legitimacy of rest: Conditions for the relief of burden in advanced dementia care-giving', *Journal of Advanced Nursing*, 66(5): 988–98. doi.org/10.1111/j.1365-2648.2010.05261.x

Dementia Care Central (no date) *Alzheimer's Life Expectancy Calculator: Introduction and Disclaimer*. Available from: www.dementiacarecentral.com/alzheimers-life-expectancy-calculator/start-page [accessed 5 September 2020].

DH (Department of Health) (UK) (2009) *Living Well with Dementia: A National Dementia Strategy*, Leeds. Available from: www.gov.uk/government/news/living-well-with-dementia-a-national-dementia-strategy [accessed 15 June 2021].

Dillman, R. (2000) 'Alzheimer disease: Epistemological lessons from history', in P. Whitehouse, K. Maurer and J. Ballenger (eds) *Concepts of Alzheimer Disease: Biological, Clinical and Cultural Perspectives*, Baltimore, MD: Johns Hopkins University Press, pp 129–57.

Driessen, A. (2019) 'A good life with dementia: Ethnographic articulations of everyday life and care in Dutch nursing homes', PhD thesis, University of Amsterdam. Available from: https://hdl.handle.net/11245.1/dd0c2b9b-348d-4de8-9747-84363846fdd0 [accessed 15 June 2021].

Dudgeon, S. (2010) *Rising Tide: The Impact of Dementia on Canadian Society: A Study*, Toronto, ON: Alzheimer Society of Canada.

Dunér, A. and Nordström, M. (2010) 'The desire for control: Negotiating the arrangement of help for older people in Sweden', *Journal of Aging Studies*, 24(4): 241–7. doi:10.1016/j.jaging.2010.05.004.

Egdell, V. (2013) 'Who cares? Managing obligation and responsibility across the changing landscapes of informal dementia care', *Ageing & Society*, 33(5): 888–907.

Egdell, V., Bond, J., Brittain, K. and Jarvis, H. (2010) 'Disparate routes through support: Negotiating the sites, stages and support of informal dementia care', *Health & Place*, 16(1): 101–7. doi:10.1016/j.healthplace.2009.09.002.

Federal/Provincial/Territorial Working Group on Home Care (1990) *Report on Home Care*, Ottawa, ON: Health and Welfare Canada.

Fernandez, J. (1972) 'Persuasions and performances: Of the beast in every body ... And the metaphors of everyman', *Daedalus*, 101(1): 39–60.

Fernandez, J. (1986) *Persuasions and Performances: The Play of Tropes in Culture*, Bloomington, IN: Indiana University Press.

Finlayson, A. (2006) ' "What's the problem?": Political theory, rhetoric and problem-setting', *Critical Review of International Social and Political Philosophy*, 9(4): 541–57.

Foucault, M. (1977) *Discipline and Punish*, London: Allen Lane.

Foucault, M. (1982a) 'Is it really important to think? An interview translated by Thomas Keenan', *Philosophy & Social Criticism*, 9(1): 30–40. doi:10.1177/019145378200900102.

Foucault, M. (1982b) 'The subject and power', *Critical Inquiry*, 8(4): 777–95.

Foucault, M. (1989a) 'Problematics', in M. Foucault and S. Lotringer (eds) *Foucault Live: Collected Interviews, 1961–1980*, New York, NY: Semiotext(e), pp 416–22.

Foucault, M. (1989b) 'The concern for the truth', in M. Foucault and S. Lotringer (eds) *Foucault Live: Collected Interviews, 1961–1980*, New York, NY: Semiotext(e), pp 455–64.

Foucault, M. (2003) *The Birth of the Clinic: An Archaeology of Medical Perception*, London: Routledge.

Franklin, U. (1999) *The Real World of Technology* (revised edn), Toronto, ON: Anansi Press.

Freeman, R. (2017) 'Care, policy, knowledge: Translating between worlds', *Sociological Review*, 65(2): 193–200.

Gadamer, H. (1976) *Philosophical Hermeneutics*, Berkeley, CA: University of California Press.

Gaines, A. and Whitehouse, P. (2006) 'Building a mystery: Alzheimer's disease, mild cognitive impairment and beyond', *Philosophy, Psychiatry, & Psychology*, 13(1): 61–74.

Garfinkel, H. (1967) *Studies in Ethnomethodology*, Cambridge: Polity Press.

Giddens, A. (1984) *The Constitution of Society: Outline of the Theory of Structuration*, Cambridge: Polity Press.

Gillies, B. (2012) 'Continuity and loss: The carer's journey through dementia', *Dementia*, 11(5): 857–76. doi.org/10.1177/1471301211421262

Glendinning, C. (2012) 'Home care in England: Markets in the context of under-funding', *Health & Social Care in the Community*, 20(3): 292–9.

Glendinning, C., Mitchell, W. and Brooks, J. (2015) 'Ambiguity in practice? Carers' roles in personalised social care in England', *Health & Social Care in the Community*, 23(1): 23–32.

Glimmerveen, L. and Nies, H. (2015) 'Integrated community-based dementia care: The geriant model', *International Journal of Integrated Care*, 15(6): e020.

Graham, J. and Bassett, R. (2006) 'Reciprocal relations: The recognition and co-construction of caring with Alzheimer's disease', *Journal of Aging Studies*, 20(4): 335–49.

Gronemeyer, R. (2017) 'The dementia-friendly community – A daring venture', in V. Rothe, R. Gronemeyer and G. Kreutzner (eds) *Staying in Life: Paving the Way to Dementia-Friendly Communities*, Bielefeld: Verlag, pp 17–41.

Gubrium, J.F. (1986) *Oldtimers and Alzheimer's: The Descriptive Organization of Senility*, Greenwich, CT: JAI Press.

Gubrium, J.F. and Järvinen, M. (2014) 'Troubles, problems, and clientization', in J.F. Gubrium and M. Järvinen (eds) *Turning Troubles into Problems: Clientization in Human Services*, Abingdon: Routledge, pp 1–14.

Haaksma, M.L., Rizzuto, D., Leoutsakos, J.-M.S., Marengoni, A., Tan, E.C.K., Olde Rikkert, M.G.M., Fratiglioni, L., Melis, R.J.F. and Calderón-Larrañaga, A. (2019) 'Predicting cognitive and functional trajectories in people with late-onset dementia: 2 population-based studies', *Journal of the American Medical Directors Association*, 20(11): 1444–50. doi.org/10.1016/j.jamda.2019.03.025

Hacking, I. (2007) 'Kinds of people: Moving targets', *Proceedings of the British Academy*, 151: 285–318.

Hammersley, M. and Atkinson, P. (2007) *Ethnography: Principles in Practice* (3rd edn), London: Routledge.

Haraway, D. (2016) *Staying with the Trouble: Making Kin in the Chthulucene*, Durham, NC: Duke University Press.

Health Council of Canada (2012) *Seniors in Need, Caregivers in Distress*, Toronto, ON. Available from: healthcouncilcanada.ca/348/ [accessed 15 June 2021].

Hollander, M.J. and Chappell, N. (2001) *Synthesis Report: Final Report of the National Evaluation of the Cost-Effectiveness of Home Care*, Victoria, BC: National Evaluation of the Cost-Effectiveness of Home Care and Health Canada, Health Transition Fund.

Hollander, M.J. and Saskatchewan Health (2006) *Home Care Program Review: Final Report*, Victoria, BC: Hollander Analytical Services.

Hollander, M.J. and Prince, M. (2008) 'Organizing healthcare delivery systems for persons with ongoing care needs and their families: A best practices framework', *Healthcare Quarterly*, 11(1): 44–54.

Hollander, M.J., Miller, J., MacAdam, M., Chappell, N. and Pedlar, D. (2009) 'Increasing value for money in the Canadian healthcare system: New findings and the case for integrated care for seniors', *Healthcare Quarterly*, 12(1): 38–47.

Holstein, M. (2000) 'Aging, culture and the framing of Alzheimer disease', in P. Whitehouse, K. Maurer and J. Ballenger (eds) *Concepts of Alzheimer Disease: Biological, Clinical and Cultural Perspectives*, Baltimore, MD: Johns Hopkins University Press, pp 158–80.

Jardine, D.W. (1992) 'The fecundity of the individual case: Considerations of the pedagogic heart of interpretive work', *Journal of Philosophy of Education*, 26(1): 51–61.

Keefe, J. (2011) *Supporting Caregivers and Caregiving in an Aging Canada*, November, Montreal, QC: Institute for Research on Public Policy.

Kelaiditi, E., Andrieu, S., Cantet, C., Vellas, B. and Cesari, M. (2016) 'Frailty index and incident mortality, hospitalization, and institutionalization in Alzheimer's disease: Data from the ICTUS study', *Journals of Gerontology Series A: Biological Sciences & Medical Sciences*, 71(4): 543–8.

Lach, H.W. and Chang, Y.P. (2007) 'Caregiver perspectives on safety in home dementia care', *Western Journal of Nursing Research*, 29(8): 993–1014.

Latimer, J. (2018) 'Repelling neoliberal world-making? How the ageing-dementia relation is reassembling the social', *Sociological Review*, 66(4): 832–56.

Latour, B. (1984) 'The powers of association', *The Sociological Review*, 32(1): 264–80. doi:10.1111/j.1467-954X.1984.tb00115.x

Latour, B. (1990) 'Technology is society made durable', in J. Law (ed) *A Sociology of Monsters: Essays on Power, Technology and Domination*, London: Routledge, pp 103–31.

Latour, B. (1991) *We Have Never Been Modern* (translated by C. Porter), Cambridge, MA: Harvard University Press.

Latour, B. (2007) 'Can we get our materialism back, please?', *Isis*, 98(1): 138–42.

Law, J. (1994) *Organizing modernity*, Oxford: Blackwell.

Law, J. (2004) *After Method: Mess in Social Science Research*, London: Routledge.

Law, J. (2008) 'On sociology and STS', *The Sociological Review*, 56(4): 623–49.

Law, J. and Mol, A. (1995) 'Notes on materiality and sociality', *Sociological Review*, 43(2): 274–94. doi.org/10.1111/j.1467-954X.1995.tb00604.x

Law, J. and Urry, J. (2004) 'Enacting the social', *Economy and Society*, 33(3): 390–410. doi:10.1080/0308514042000225716.

Law, J., Afdal, G., Asdal, K., Lin, W., Moser, I. and Singleton, V. (2013) 'Modes of syncretism: Notes on noncoherence', *Common Knowledge*, 20(1): 172–92.

Le Couteur, D.G., Doust, J., Creasey, H. and Brayne, C. (2013) 'Political drive to screen for pre-dementia: Not evidence based and ignores the harms of diagnosis', *BMJ*, 347: f5125. doi.org/10.1136/bmj.f5125

Lilly, M., Robinson, C., Holtzman, S. and Bottorff, J. (2012) 'Can we move beyond burden and burnout to support the health and wellness of family caregivers to persons with dementia? Evidence from British Columbia, Canada', *Health and Social Care in the Community*, 20(1): 103–12.

Liveng, A. (2011) 'The vulnerable elderly's need for recognizing relationships – A challenge to Danish home-based care', *Journal of Social Work Practice*, 25(3): 271–83.

Lloyd, B.T. and Stirling, C. (2011) 'Ambiguous gain: Uncertain benefits of service use for dementia carers', *Sociology of Health & Illness*, 33(6): 899–913.

Lloyd, L. (2012) *Health and Care in Ageing Societies: A New International Approach*, Bristol: Policy Press.

Lock, M. (2013) *The Alzheimer Conundrum: Entanglements of Dementia and Aging*, Princeton, NJ: Princeton University Press.

López, D. (2015) 'Little arrangements that matter: Rethinking autonomy-enabling innovations for later life', *Technological Forecasting & Social Change*, 93: 91–101.

Low, L., White, F., Jeon, Y., Gresham, M. and Brodaty, H. (2013) 'Desired characteristics and outcomes of community care services for persons with dementia: What is important according to clients, service providers and policy?', *Australasian Journal on Ageing*, 32(2): 91–6.

Lymbery, M. (2010) 'A new vision for adult social care? Continuities and change in the care of older people', *Critical Social Policy*, 30(1): 5–26.

Lyons, K.S. and Zarit, S.H. (1999) 'Formal and informal support: The great divide', *International Journal of Geriatric Psychiatry*, 14(3): 183–96.

MacAdam, M. (2009) *Moving toward Health Services Integration: Provincial Progress in System Change for Seniors*, Toronto, ON: Canadian Policy Research Networks.

Macdonald, M., Lang, A., Storch, J., Stevenson, L., Donaldson, S., Barber, T. and Iaboni, K. (2013) 'Home care safety markers: A scoping review', *Home Health Care Services Quarterly*, 32(2): 126–48. doi:10.1080/01621424.2013.783523.

Marres, N., Guggenheim, M. and Wilkie, A. (2018) 'From performance to inventing the social', in N. Marres, M. Guggenheim and A. Wilkie (eds) *Inventing the Social*, Manchester: Mattering Press, pp 17–37.

May, C. (2012) 'Illness is a plural: Homecare, governmentality and reframing the work of patienthood', in C. Ceci, K. Björnsdóttir and M.E. Purkis (eds) *Perspectives on Care at Home for Older People*, London: Routledge, pp ix–xiii.

McGranahan, C. (2014) 'What is ethnography? Teaching ethnographic sensibilities without fieldwork', *Teaching Anthropology*, 4: 23–36. doi:10.22582/ta.v4i1.421.

Mohide, E., Torrance, G., Streiner, D., Pringle, D. and Gilbert, R. (1988) 'Measuring the wellbeing of family caregivers using the time trade-off technique', *Journal of Clinical Epidemiology*, 41(5): 475–82.

Moise, P., Schwarzinger, M., Um, M. and the Dementia Experts' Group (2004) *Dementia Care in 9 OECD Countries: A Comparative Analysis*, Paris: OECD. Available from: www.oecd.org/dataoecd/10/52/33661491.pdf [accessed 2 June 2021].

Mol, A. (2002) *The Body Multiple: Ontology in Medical Practice*, London: Duke University Press.

Mol, A. (2008) *The Logic of Care: Health and the Problem of Patient Choice*, London: Routledge.

Mol, A. and Law, J. (2002) 'Complexities: An introduction', in J. Law and A. Mol (eds) *Complexities: Social Studies of Knowledge Practices*, Durham, NC: Duke University Press, pp 1–22.

Mol, A., Moser, I. and Pols, J. (2010) 'Care: Putting practice into theory', in A. Mol, I. Moser and J. Pols (eds) *Care in Practice: On Tinkering in Clinics, Homes and Farms*, Bielefeld: Transcript, pp 7–25.

Moreira, T. (2017) *Science, Technology and the Ageing Society*, Abingdon: Routledge.

Moreira, T. and Palladino, P. (2008) 'Squaring the curve: The anatomo-politics of ageing, life and death', *Body & Society*, 14(3), 21–47. doi:10.1177/1357034X08093571.

Moser, I. (2005) 'On becoming disabled and articulating alternatives: The multiple modes of ordering disability and their interferences', *Cultural Studies*, 19(6): 667–700.

Moser, I. (2008) 'Making Alzheimer's disease matter: Enacting, interfering and doing politics of nature', *Geoforum*, 39(1): 98–110.

Moser, I. (2010) 'Perhaps tears should not be counted but wiped away: On quality and improvement in dementia care', in A. Mol, I. Moser and J. Pols (eds) *Care in Practice: On Tinkering in Clinics, Homes and Farms*, London: Transaction Publishers, pp 277–300.

Moser, I. (2011) 'Dementia and the limits to life: Anthropological sensibilities, STS interferences, and possibilities for action in care', *Science, Technology & Human Values*, 36(5): 704–22.

National Conference on Home Care (1998) *Proceedings*, Ottawa, ON: Health Canada.

NIA (National Institute on Ageing) (2019) *Enabling the Future Provision of Long-Term Care in Canada*, White Paper, Toronto, ON. Available from: https://static1.squarespace.com/static/5c2fa7b03917eed9b5a436d8/t/5d9de15a38dca21e46009548/1570627931078/Enabling+the+Future+Provision+of+Long-Term+Care+in+Canada.pdf [accessed 15 June 2021].

Nicolini, D. (2012) *Practice Theory, Work, and Organization: An Introduction*, Oxford: Oxford University Press.

Nies, H., Meerveld, J. and Denis, R. (2009) 'Dementia care: Linear links and networks', *HealthcarePapers*, 10(1): 34–43.

Nocek, A.J. (2018) 'On the risk of Gaia for an ecology of practices', *Substance: A Review of Theory & Literary Criticism*, 47(1): 96–111.

Norton, S., Matthews, F. E. and Brayne, C. (2013) 'A commentary on studies presenting projections of the future prevalence of dementia', *BMC Public Health*, 13(1): 1–5. doi.org/10.1186/1471-2458-13-1

OECD (Organisation for Economic Co-operation and Development) (2015) *Addressing Dementia: The OECD Response*, Paris: OECD Publishing.

OECD (2018) *Renewing Priority for Dementia: Where Do We Stand?*, Paris: OECD Publishing.

Ong, A. (2006) 'Mutations in citizenship', *Theory, Culture & Society*, 23(2–3): 499–505. doi.org/10.1177/0263276406064831

Open Learn (no date) 'Dementia Awareness: What is dementia, and how can we reduce the risk?'. Available from: www.open.edu/openlearn/health-sports-psychology/mental-health/dementia-awareness-what-dementia-and-how-can-we-reduce-the-risk [accessed 5 September 2020].

O'Shea, E., Timmons, S., O'Shea, E. and Irving, K. (2019) 'Multiple stakeholders' perspectives on respite service access for people with dementia and their carers', *Gerontologist*, 59(5): e490–e500.

O'Shea, E., Timmons, S., O'Shea, E., Fox, S. and Irving, K. (2017) 'Key stakeholders' experiences of respite services for people with dementia and their perspectives on respite service development: A qualitative systematic review', *BMC Geriatrics*, 17: 1–14. doi:10.1186/s12877-017-0676-0.

Palsson, G. (1994) 'Enskilment at sea', *Man*, 29(4): 901–27.

Parent, K. and Anderson, M. (1999) *CARP's Report Card on Home Care in Canada, 1999*, Toronto, ON: Canadian Association of Retired Persons (CARP).

Parker, M. (2015) 'Organization and philosophy: Vision and division', in R. Mir, H. Willmott and M. Greenwood (eds) *The Routledge Companion to Philosophy in Organization Studies*, Abingdon: Routledge, pp 491–8.

Peel, E. (2014) ' "The living death of Alzheimer's" versus "Take a walk to keep dementia at bay": Representations of dementia in print media and carer discourse', *Sociology of Health & Illness*, 36(6): 885–901. doi.org/10.1111/1467-9566.12122

PHAC (Public Health Agency of Canada) (2019) *A Dementia Strategy for Canada: Together We Aspire*, Ottawa, ON: PHAC. Available from: https://www.canada.ca/en/public-health/services/publications/diseases-conditions/dementia-strategy.html [accessed 15 June 2021].

Pols, J. (2010) 'Bringing bodies – and health care – back in: Exploring practical knowledge for living with chronic disease', *Medische Antropologie*, 22(2): 413–27.

Pols, J. (2012) *Care at a Distance: On the Closeness of Technology*, Amsterdam: Amsterdam University Press.

Pols, J. (2014) 'Knowing patients: Turning patient knowledge into science', *Science, Technology, & Human Values*, 39(1): 73–97.

Pols, J. (2018) 'Care, everyday life, and aesthetic values: About the study of specificities', in J. Brouwer and S. van Tuinen (eds) *To Mind is to Care*, Rotterdam, NL: V2, pp 42–61.

Portacolone, E., Berridge, C., Johnson, J.K. and Schicktanz, S. (2014) 'Time to reinvent the science of dementia: The need for care and social integration', *Aging & Mental Health*, 18(3): 269–75.

Purkis, M.E. (2003) 'Moving nursing practice: Integrating theory and method', in J. Latimer (ed) *Advanced Qualitative Research for Nursing*, London: Blackwell Science, pp 32–50.

Purkis, M.E. and Ceci, C. (2015) 'Problematizing care burden research', *Ageing & Society*, 35(7): 1410–28.

Purkis, M.E., Ceci, C. and Björnsdóttir, K. (2008) 'Patching up the holes: Analysing the work of home care', *Canadian Journal of Public Health*, 99(S2): S27–S32

Rabinow, P. (2005) 'Midst anthropology's problems', in A. Ong and S. Collier (eds) *Global Assemblages: Technology, Politics and Ethics as Anthropological Problems*, Malden, MA: Blackwell Publishing, pp 40–53.

Richards, M. and Brayne, C. (2010) 'What do we mean by Alzheimer's disease?', *BMJ*, 341: c4670.

Rose, N. and Miller, P. (2010) 'Political power beyond the State: Problematics of government', *The British Journal of Sociology*, 61(1): 271–303. doi:10.1111/j.1468-4446.2009.01247.x

Rossiter, K., Kontos, P., Colantonio, A., Gilbert, J., Gray, J. and Keightley, M. (2008) 'Staging data: Theatre as a tool for analysis and knowledge transfer in health research', *Social Science & Medicine*, 66(1): 130–46. doi:10.1016/j.socscimed.2007.07.021

Rostgaard, T., Timonen, V. and Glendinning, C. (2012) 'Guest Editorial: Reforming home care in ageing societies', *Health & Social Care in the Community*, 20(3): 225–7. doi:10.1111/j.1365-2524.2012.01071.x

Sadler, E. and McKevitt, C. (2013) '"Expert carers": An emergent normative model of the caregiver', *Social Theory & Health*, 11: 40–58.

Samus, Q.M., Black, B.S., Bovenkamp, D., Buckley, M., Callahan, C., Davis, K., Gitlin, L.N., Hodgson, N., Johnston, D., Kales, H.C., Karel, M., Kenney, J.J., Ling, S.M., Panchal, M., Reuland, M., Willink, A. and Lyketsos, C.G. (2018) 'Home is where the future is: The BrightFocus Foundation consensus panel on dementia care', *Alzheimer's & Dementia: The Journal of The Alzheimer's Association*, 14(1): 104–14.

Savransky, M. (2018) 'The social and its problems: On problematic sociology', in N. Marres, M. Guggenheim and A. Wilkie (eds) *Inventing the Social*, Manchester: Mattering Press, pp 212–33.

Savransky, M. and Stengers, I. (2018) 'Relearning the art of paying attention: A conversation', *SubStance #145*, 47(1): 130–45.

Schillmeier, M. (2017) 'The cosmopolitics of situated care', *Sociological Review*, 65(2): 55–70.

Schutz, A. (1944) 'The stranger: An essay in social psychology', *The American Journal of Sociology*, 49(6): 499–507.

Schutz, A. (1946) 'The well-informed citizen: An essay on the social distribution of knowledge', *Social Research*, 13(4): 463–78.

Simonet, D. (2008) 'The new public management theory and European health-care reforms', *Canadian Public Administration*, 51(4): 617–35.

Sims-Gould, J. and Martin-Matthews, A. (2010) 'We share the care: Family caregivers' experiences of their older relative receiving home support services', *Health and Social Care in the Community*, 18(4): 415–23.

Somers, M.R. (2008) *Genealogies of Citizenship: Markets, Statelessness, and the Right to Have Rights*, Cambridge: Cambridge University Press.

Speechley, M., DeForge, R.T., Ward-Griffin, C., Marlatt, N.M. and Gutmanis, I. (2015) 'Creating an ethnodrama to catalyze dialogue in home-based dementia care', *Qualitative Health Research*, 25(11): 1551–9. doi:10.1177/1049732315609572

Spoelstra, S. (2005) 'Robert Cooper: Beyond organization', *Sociological Review Monograph*, 53(2): 106–19.

Stajduhar, K., Funk, L., Jakobsson, E. and Öhlén, J. (2010) 'A critical analysis of health promotion and "empowerment" in the context of palliative family care-giving', *Nursing Inquiry*, 17(3): 221–30. doi:10.1111/j.1440-1800.2009.00483.x

St-Amant, O., Ward-Griffin, C., DeForge, R.T., Oudshoorn, A., McWilliam, C., Forbes, D., Kloseck, M. and Hall, J. (2012) 'Making care decisions in home-based dementia care: Why context matters', *Canadian Journal on Aging*, 31(4): 423–34.

Star, S.L. (1990) 'Power, technology and the phenomenology of conventions: On being allergic to onions', *The Sociological Review*, 38(1): 26–56.

Starobinski, J. (1975) 'The inside and the outside', *The Hudson Review*, 28(3): 333–51.

Stengers, I. (2005a) 'Introductory notes on an ecology of practices', *Cultural Studies Review*, 11(1): 183–96.

Stengers, I. (2005b) 'The cosmopolitical proposal', in B. Latour and P. Weibel (eds) *Making Things Public: Atmospheres of Democracy*, Cambridge, MA: MIT Press, pp 994–1003.

Stengers, I. (2015 [2009]) *In Catastrophic Times: Resisting the Coming Barbarism* (translated by A. Goffey), Lüneburg: Meson Press [Open Humanities Press].

Stengers, I. (2017) 'The insistence of possibles: Towards a speculative pragmatism', *Parse*, 7, Autumn. Available from: https://parsejournal.com/article/the-insistence-of-possibles%E2%80%A8-towards-a-speculative-pragmatism/ [accessed 2 June 2021].

Stengers, I. (2018) 'Postlude', *SubStance #145*, 47(1): 146–55.

Stengers, I. (2019) 'Comparison as a matter of concern', *Common Knowledge*, 25 (1–3): 176–91.

Stephan, A., Bieber, A., Hopper, L., Joyce, R., Irving, K., Zanetti, O., Portolani, E., Kerpershoek, L., Verhey, F., de Vugt, M., Wolfs, C., Eriksen, S., Røsvik, J., Marques, M.J., Gonçalves-Pereira, M., Sjölund, B.M., Jelley, H., Woods, B. and Meyer, G. (2018) 'Barriers and facilitators to the access to and use of formal dementia care: Findings of a focus group study with people with dementia, informal carers and health and social care professionals in eight European countries', *BMC Geriatrics*, 18(1): 131.

Stevenson, M., McDowell, M.E. and Taylor, B.J. (2018) 'Concepts for communication about risk in dementia care: A review of the literature', *Dementia*, 17(3): 359–90.

Stirling, C.M., Dwan, C.A. and McKenzie, A.R. (2014) 'Why carers use adult day respite: A mixed method case study', *BMC Health Services Research*, 14: 245.

Straßheim, J. (2016) 'Type and spontaneity: Beyond Alfred Schutz's theory of the social world', *Human Studies*, 39(4): 493–512.

Taylor, J., Namey, E., Carrington Johnson, A. and Guest, G. (2017) 'Beyond the page: A process review of using ethnodrama to disseminate research findings', *Journal of Health Communication*, 22(6): 532–44. doi:10.1080/10810730.2017.1317303

Thygesen, H. and Moser, I. (2010) 'Technology and good dementia care: An argument for an ethics-in-practice-approach', in M. Schillmeyer and M. Domenech (eds) *New Technologies and Emerging Spaces of Care*, London: Ashgate, pp 129–47.

Tsing, A. (2015) *The Mushroom at the End of the World: On the Possibility of Life in Capitalist Ruins*, Princeton, NJ: Princeton University Press.

Tufte, P. and Dahl, H.M. (2016) 'Navigating the field of temporally framed care in the Danish home care sector', *Sociology of Health & Illness*, 38(1): 109–22.

Twigg, J. (1989) 'Models of carers: How do social care agencies conceptualise their relationship with informal carers?', *Journal of Social Policy*, 18(1): 53–66.

Ulmanen, P. and Szebehely, M. (2015) 'From the state to the family or to the market? Consequences of reduced residential eldercare in Sweden', *International Journal of Social Welfare*, 24(1): 81–92.

Waldorff, F., Buss, D., Eckermann, A., Rasmussen, M., Keiding, N., Rishøj, S., Siersma, V., Sørensen. J., Sørensen, L.V., Vogel, A. and Waldemar, G. (2012) 'Efficacy of psychosocial intervention in patients with mild Alzheimer's disease: The multicentre, rater blinded, randomised Danish Alzheimer intervention study (DAISY)', *BMJ*, 345: e4693. doi:10.1136/bmj.e4693

Walsh, S., O'Shea, E., Pierse, T., Kennelly, B., Keogh, F. and Doherty, E. (2020) 'Public preferences for home care services for people with dementia: A discrete choice experiment on personhood', *Social Science & Medicine*, 245: 112675. doi:10.1016/j.socscimed.2019.112675.

Ward-Griffin, C. and McKeever, P. (2000) 'Relationships between nurses and family caregivers: Partners in care?', *Advances in Nursing Science*, 22(3): 89–103.

Whitehouse, P. J. and George, D. (2008) *The Myth of Alzheimer's: What You Aren't Being Told about Today's Most Dreaded Diagnosis*, New York, NY: St Martin's Griffin.

Wiles, J. (2003) 'Informal caregivers' experiences of formal support in a changing context', *Health & Social Care in the Community*, 11(3): 189–207.

Wilkinson, S. (2016) 'Analysing focus group data', in D. Silverman (ed) *Qualitative Research* (4th edn), London: SAGE Publications Ltd, pp 83–98.

Williams, A.P., Lum, J., Deber, R., Montgomery, R., Kuluski, K., Peckham, A., Watkins, J., Williams, A., Ying, A. and Zhu, L. (2009) 'Aging at home: Integrating community-based care for older persons', *HealthcarePapers*, 10(1): 8–21.

Winthereik, B.R. and Verran, H. (2012) 'Ethnographic stories as generalizations that intervene', *Science Studies*, 25(1): 37–51.

WHO (World Health Organization) (2012) *Dementia: A Public Health Priority*, Geneva. Available from: www.who.int/mental_health/publications/dementia_report_2012/en/ [accessed 2 June 2021].

WHO (2018) *Meeting on the Implementation of the Global Action Plan on the Public Health Response to Dementia 2017–2025*, Geneva. Available from: www.who.int/mental_health/neurology/dementia/action_plan_2017_2025/en/ [accessed 2 June 2021].

Wu, Y.-T., Fratiglioni, L., Matthews, F.E., Lobo, A., Breteler, M. M.B., Skoog, I. and Brayne, C. (2016) 'Dementia in western Europe: Epidemiological evidence and implications for policy making', *The Lancet Neurology*, 15(1): 116–24.

Yang, J. (2015) 'Dementia: A private tragedy looms as a public catastrophe worldwide', *Toronto Star*, 22 March. Available from: www.thestar.com/news/world/2015/03/22/dementia-a-private-tragedy-looms-as-a-public-catastrophe-worldwide.html?rf [accessed 2 July 2021].

Zarit, S. H. and Femia, E. (2008) 'A future for family care and dementia intervention research? Challenges and strategies', *Aging & Mental Health*, 12(1): 5–13.

Zarit, S.H., Reeves, K.E. and Bach-Peterson, J. (1980) 'Relatives of the impaired elderly: Correlates of feelings of burden', *Gerontologist*, 20(6): 649–55.

Zarit, S.H., Gaugler, J.E. and Jarrott, S.E. (1999) 'Useful services for families: Research findings and directions', *International Journal of Geriatric Psychiatry*, 14(3): 165–81.

Index